THE
TUI NA
MANUAL

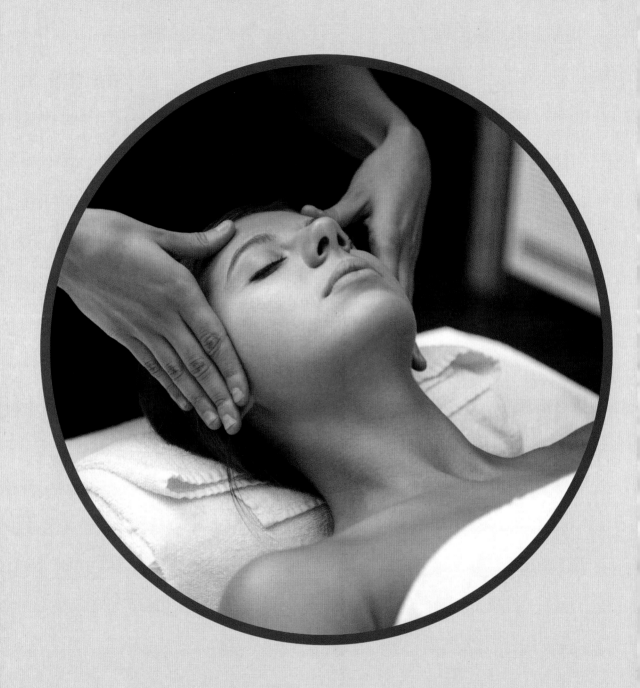

MARIA MERCATI

THE **TUI NA** MANUAL

CHINESE MASSAGE TO AWAKEN BODY AND MIND

Healing Arts Press
Rochester, Vermont • Toronto, Canada

To my loving family:
Trevor, Gisela, Gina, Graham, and Danella

Healing Arts Press
One Park Street
Rochester, Vermont 05767
www.HealingArtsPress.com

Healing Arts Press is a division of Inner Traditions International

First published in the United Kingdom in 1997 by Gaia Books Limited under the title
Step-by-Step Tui Na: Massage to Awaken Body and Mind
First U.S. edition published in 1997 by Healing Arts Press under the title *The Handbook
    of Chinese Massage: Tui Na Techniques to Awaken Body and Mind*
Second U.S. edition published in 2018 by Healing Arts Press under the title *The Tui Na
    Manual: Chinese Massage to Awaken Body and Mind*

Note to the reader: *This book is intended as an informational guide. The remedies, approaches,
and techniques described herein are meant to supplement, and not to be a substitute for,
professional medical care or treatment. They should not be used to treat a serious ailment
without prior consultation with a qualified health care professional.*

Library of Congress Cataloging-in-Publication Data
Names: Mercati, Maria. author.
Title: The Tui Na manual : Chinese massage to awaken body and mind / Maria Mercati.
Other titles: Handbook of Chinese massage
Description: Second U.S. edition. | Rochester, Vermont : Healing Arts Press, 2018. | Revision
    of: Handbook of Chinese massage. 1997. | Includes bibliographical references and index.
Identifiers: LCCN 2018003358 (print) | LCCN 2018004238 (e-book) |
    ISBN 9781620557495 (paperback) | ISBN 9781620557501 (e-book)
Subjects: LCSH: Massage—China—Handbooks, manuals, etc. | BISAC: HEALTH & FITNESS /
    Massage & Reflexotherapy. | BODY, MIND & SPIRIT / Healing / Energy (Chi Kung, Reiki,
    Polarity). | MEDICAL / Allied Health Services / Massage Therapy.
Classification: LCC RM723.C5 M47 2018 (print) | LCC RM723.C5 (e-book) |
    DDC 615.8/22—dc23
LC record available at https://lccn.loc.gov/2018003358

Printed and bound in China

10 9 8 7 6 5 4 3 2 1

CONTENTS

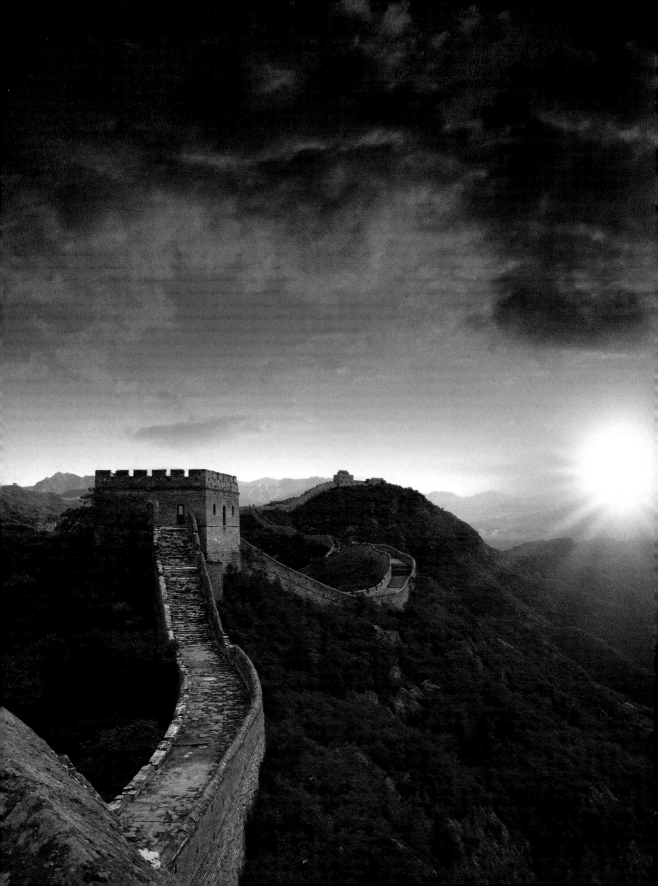

A NOTE FROM THE AUTHOR

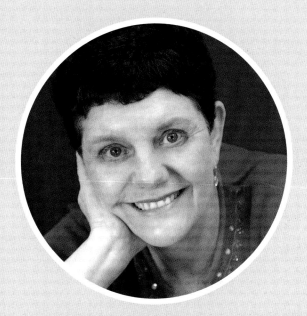

I discovered Tui Na during my own personal quest for a therapy to relieve crippling pain. As a child I suffered from a degenerative disease that affected my hip. While living in Indonesia for four years, I discovered the healing powers of deep oriental massage, and trained as a massage therapist. As the years went by, standing and walking even for short distances caused me pain. In 1987, Western medicine could only offer me painkillers and a hip replacement operation. But instead of going to hospital for surgery, I travelled to China to learn Tui Na. The skilful, patient doctors of traditional medicine gave me the treatment and tuition that I needed and opened a wonderful new chapter in my life.

At that time, few people in the West had heard of Tui Na, although acupuncture and herbal medicine were available. So extraordinary was Tui Na's effect on me, it became my mission in life to bring it within the reach of everyone in the West. I studied, worked and travelled back to China time and again to learn Tui Na and acupuncture from Chinese doctors in hospitals and clinics in Shanghai, Weihai, Xi'an, Beijing and Jinan.

In response to a growing interest in Tui Na and acupuncture, I established the teaching side of the BODYHARMONICS® Centre, where we run regular training courses. Over the decades, I have trained hundreds of students in Tui Na and acupuncture (www.bodyharmonics.co.uk).

I have treated many people with disabling conditions where other forms of medicine could do little to help and have found that there is a real alternative to living on painkillers or having surgery. Tui Na has changed my life and the lives of many of my patients, and also my students and their patients. I hope that it can do the same for you.

M. B. Mercati.

AUTHOR'S ACKNOWLEDGEMENTS

I owe a debt of gratitude to the Chinese doctors of the traditional Chinese hospitals of Shanghai, Weihai, Xi'an and Jinan, who have most generously and patiently taught me the theory and practice of Tui Na.

My thanks also go to my husband Trevor for the enjoyable hours of discussion and brainstorming involved in preparing this book, and to my daughters Gisela, Gina and Danella, my son Graham, Jamie Dawkins, Neal Wickens and my grandchildren Oscar, Claudia and Rosa for patiently and skilfully modelling for most of the photographs and being excellent ambassadors for Tui Na. I would like to give a special thanks to Darren Tucker for patiently correcting all qi-points and meridians.

HOW TO USE THIS BOOK

The Tui Na Manual provides a comprehensive introduction to the use of this ancient healing art of deep massage and manipulation. Accessible for readers who have no previous experience of massage therapies, its clear approach is also valuable for those trained in other forms of bodywork, or in traditional Chinese medicine.

Chapters 1 and 2 describe the unique features of Tui Na and explain its roots in the 4,000-year-old system of traditional Chinese medicine. These chapters give important background information for the more practical techniques that follow in the remaining chapters.

Chapter 3 uses illustrations and descriptions to show the energy pathways in the body, and the points where this energy can be manipulated. You need to familiarize yourself with these and practise the Tui Na techniques for soft tissue massage and joint manipulations described in chapter 4, before going on to giving the treatments described in the final two chapters.

The whole-body routine in chapter 5 is a unique holistic treatment, developed by the author. In China, there is no specific routine; only techniques for healthcare and health conditions.

Focusing on each part of the body in turn, it restores balance in the body's energies, for health and well-being in body, mind and spirit. Once you have mastered the techniques and learned how to give the whole-body treatment, you can modify it, if necessary, to meet your partner's needs.

Chapter 6 presents treatments for a variety of common conditions and ailments. One section is devoted to sports injuries, such as sprains and muscle strains, which can be treated very successfully using Tui Na. There are also treatments appropriate for infants, adolescents and the elderly.

Tui Na is part of a medical system of healing, and for accuracy its techniques and applications have to be explained using medical anatomical terms. These are explained in the Appendix, which includes diagrams of the bones and muscles in the body, and the Glossary.

Many anatomical terms, such as the names of the organs of the body, and bodily fluids, such as blood or phlegm, have a wider meaning in Chinese medicine than they do in the West (see page 18), and this meaning is implicit in the use of these terms throughout this book.

NOTE ON SAFETY

The techniques and treatments in this book are to be used at the reader's sole discretion and risk. Always observe the cautions given, and consult a doctor if you are in any doubt about a medical condition.

Tui Na is very safe when performed according to the advice given in this book. One of its major applications is in relieving pain, but it can also be used to treat a wide range of common ailments. As with any form of deep massage, there are certain contraindications, which are given on page 62. Some of the treatments should not be used during pregnancy; wherever this is the case, the treatments are highlighted with a caution.

THE PROMISE OF TUI NA

Tui Na massage is one of the ancient healing arts of traditional Chinese medicine (also referred to in this book as TCM), along with acupuncture and herbal medicine. The earliest writings on Chinese medicine are in the Nei Ching, *translated as* The Yellow Emperor's Classic of Internal Medicine, *dating back to around 2300* BCE. *The* Nei Ching, *a monumental treatise, includes several chapters on massage.*

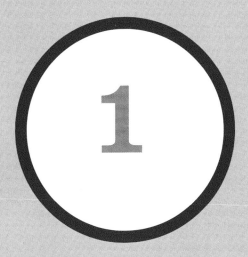

Although Tui Na has been practised in China for more than 4,000 years, and is available today in many hospitals and clinics throughout that country, it is only now becoming known in the West. The name, Tui Na, comes from Chinese and conveys the vigorous nature of this hands-on healing system: 'Tui' means 'push' and 'Na' means 'grasp'. The Chinese script on the opposite page means Tui Na. Tui Na as practised in China treats conditions that in the West would require an osteopath, chiropractor, physiotherapist or sports therapist. Unlike these techniques, it works not only on the muscles and joints but also at a deeper level, affecting the flow of vital life energy in the body. In Chinese theory, this life energy is called 'qi' (pronounced 'chee'). Qi is the activating energy for all life processes. In the body, qi flows in clearly defined energy currents. These are called 'meridians' or 'channels' and they carry qi to all the organs and tissues of the body. The concept of qi and the meridian system is explained in more detail in chapters 2 and 3.

Tui Na massage applies pressure to the meridians and specific points on them called 'qi-points' or acupressure points. Acupuncturists call them 'acupoints'. Tui Na affects the flow of qi so that it moves freely, evenly and powerfully around the body. The distribution and intensity of qi within your body have profound effects on all aspects of your well-being – the emotional, intellectual and spiritual, as well as the physical. Chinese medicine views all disease as caused by weakness, imbalances and blockages in the flow of qi. When your qi-flow is balanced you feel full of energy, stress-free and able to cope with the pressures of daily life. You will be free from stiffness, aches and pains, and so full of vitality that you 'sparkle'. Hopefully most of us have experienced this wonderful feeling of well-being at some point in our lives. The secret of Chinese medicine is how to maintain it.

FACTORS AFFECTING QI-FLOW

Many physical and emotional factors disturb the flow of qi in the body, and these can be divided into two broad categories: excesses or deficiencies. Excesses, common in the Western lifestyle, include stress, overwork and general overindulgence, while common deficiencies are poor diet, insufficient exercise and lack of sleep. Pressure to cope with deadlines, be successful and achieve status within a peer group can create an imbalance between the output necessary to reach your goals and the input that will restore mind and body. Such an imbalance can lead to overconsumption of sugar-rich foods and stimulants such as coffee or fizzy drinks to enhance the 'output'. Alcohol, recreational drugs and even too much sex can be substitutes for relaxation.

In the Chinese view, extreme emotions negatively affect organ function and qi balance throughout the body. It's healthy to experience emotion, but too much excitement can overstimulate the flow of qi, causing feelings of restlessness and insomnia, for example, while holding on to worry, feelings of anger and frustration can lead to depression. These relationships are explained in chapter 2.

All excesses and deficiencies are disruptive to the qi-balancing process. In contrast, good sleep, relaxation, regular exercise, good diet and happy relationships all promote and strengthen the smooth flow of qi.

SHIATSU – A DERIVATIVE OF TUI NA

Around 1,000 years ago Tui Na was introduced into Japan, where it was modified to become what is now known as Shiatsu. Both systems aim to balance the flow of qi throughout the body and the meridians. Shiatsu uses relatively few techniques that apply slow and sustained static pressure, whereas Tui Na uses a wide range of vigorous and penetrating techniques, such as squeezing, pushing, kneading and manipulation, to achieve improved energy flow in the tissues.

Although the ideal is to create balance and harmony in every aspect of our lives, this can be extremely difficult to maintain. Tui Na is a powerful way of helping to achieve that balance and harmony.

HEALING POWERS IN PRACTICE

Tui Na works holistically to promote qi-flow throughout the body. A practitioner will ask questions about a patient's health and lifestyle, while observing their physical condition. This will reveal their qi, jing, shen, blood, body fluid and yin/yang status (see pages 16–17) so that appropriate meridians and qi-points can be the focus of the Tui Na treatment.

For musculoskeletal pain, the practitioner palpates the painful areas to identify the most affected meridians and the qi-points that must be used for the treatment. During the massage, feedback from the patient on what feels good, or painful, guides the practitioner to the qi-points and the amount of pressure to use.

TUI NA FOR EVERYONE

Throughout China, Tui Na is practised from cradle to old age. Babies and younger children do not have fully mature meridian systems, and additional points and techniques have been developed for them. It is a very safe therapy: if pressure is applied in the wrong place, for example, it may not achieve the desired results but no harm will be done. Massage treatment may not be suitable, however, for people with certain serious health conditions (see page 62 for contraindications).

In this book, wherever a treatment described is contraindicated for certain conditions, it carries a caution note.

Tui Na's unique techniques that focus on the meridians and specific qi-points make it particularly effective for treating muscle and joint pain resulting from sports injury, wear and tear, arthritis or any other cause. All massage therapies aid relaxation, but, in addition to relaxing the muscles, Tui Na also manipulates qi-flow in the meridians and their qi-points to balance the underlying energetics of the body to achieve healing and regeneration.

Tui Na has the power to boost energy where there is qi and blood deficiency, as well as to clear blockages that have caused qi and blood stagnation.

Tui Na is excellent for a variety of ailments and conditions, including stress-related disorders. It also boosts vitality and well-being, which in turn stimulates the immune system and improves general health. This book shows you useful techniques to help relieve pain and the symptoms of many common ailments. However, it does not replace professional healthcare and you should always consult a qualified practitioner or doctor if symptoms persist.

A TUI NA TREATMENT

The massage is best given through cotton clothing to facilitate its effectiveness. Traditional Tui Na techniques do not require the use of oils. The room should be warm. During the massage, the receiver either sits on an upright chair or lies on a massage couch, depending on which part of the body is being treated. Chapter 5, page 82, explains preparing for treatment in more detail.

To be effective, many Tui Na techniques are vigorous and need to be applied with reasonable pressure. If there is a significant problem, they will initially feel slightly uncomfortable or even painful. This discomfort will ease as the massage progresses and more qi and blood are brought to the affected area to remove stagnation. After the treatment, the tissues and muscles should feel relaxed, invigorated and less painful.

Uniquely, Tui Na, with its focus on meridians and qi-points, stimulates the entire musculoskeletal system, while also supporting healthy function of all the internal organs. Since Tui Na rebalances qi-flow,

the mind and the emotions will also be affected. In most cases, a Tui Na treatment will leave the recipient feeling rejuvenated and relaxed. The massage can sometimes release blocked emotions, with the effect that the receiver may feel 'weepy' or emotional after the treatment. If this should happen, the Chinese way is to acknowledge these emotions, and then to let them go.

This book explains the Chinese view of health and the causes of disease, and shows you how to give a holistic whole-body Tui Na treatment to a partner, as well as techniques for treating common ailments and conditions. Chapter 2 explains the theories of traditional Chinese medicine and how these differ from the Western medical approach. In Chapter 3, the twelve meridians and their energetic relationships (and the two 'extraordinary' ones used in Tui Na) are illustrated and explained, with clear descriptions to enable you to find the qi-points – the points on the meridians where qi can be most easily manipulated.

Chapter 4 concentrates on the basic techniques used in Tui Na massage. It starts with soft tissue techniques: applying either static pressure or pressure with movement to the body tissues, in order to improve qi and blood flow to strengthen the body and remove stagnation. These soft tissue techniques include pulling, pushing, squeezing and kneading. The second part of chapter 4 deals with joint manipulation techniques, which are similar to those used in osteopathy and chiropractice but give the added benefit of regulating qi and blood flow. You will need to familiarize yourself with all the techniques so that you can apply them when they are used in the treatments in chapters 5 and 6.

The whole-body routine presented in chapter 5 provides step-by-step instructions for giving a Tui Na treatment to a partner. The routine starts with treatments on the neck and shoulders, and then works on the arms, back, legs and feet, ending with Tui Na on the trunk and head.

One of the strengths of Tui Na is its application to muscle and joint injury, as described in chapter 6. This chapter also presents treatments for some common ailments and conditions, and Tui Na that is particularly suitable for infants, adolescents and the elderly. There are some techniques and qi-points that you can use effectively on yourself. These are described in a self-massage routine, which, used daily, will increase your energy levels, boost your immune system and promote health and well-being.

TRADITIONAL CHINESE MEDICINE

To understand the healing powers of Tui Na, it's important to understand how Chinese medical theory views the causes of ill health and provides a system for its accurate diagnosis and treatment.

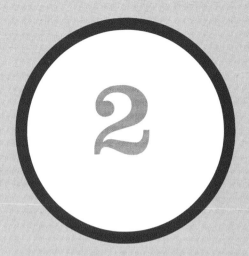

On the journey from health to disease a variety of symptoms will appear over a period of time. At first they are very subtle, but are nevertheless warning signs telling us that our health is at risk. Do you ever experience extreme tiredness, lack of energy, aches and pains, bloating after eating, headaches, poor sleep, feeling hot and sweaty or always cold, or feeling stressed and irritable? All these symptoms are an early indication of disturbances in the body's internal balance. Traditional Chinese medicine (TCM) provides you with the knowledge to understand them.

The fundamental substances

In traditional Chinese medicine, the fundamental 'five substances' are qi, jing, shen, blood and body fluids. Of these, qi, jing and shen are energetic in nature rather than material substances like blood and body fluids.

Light, heat, magnetism and electricity are all familiar examples of energy that are recognized through their effects. Substances, as such, have a physical form and can be detected by our sense of touch as well as through observation. In Western medical science, the most fundamental energy is none of the aforementioned examples but rather a form of energy that results from chemical reactions taking place within our bodies. This chemical energy comes from the food we eat, the liquids we drink and oxygen in the air we breathe, but it requires a complex series of chemical reactions to release it.

THE ENERGETIC SUBSTANCES – QI, JING AND SHEN

Qi, jing and shen are regarded as the 'Three Treasures' in TCM because each is essential for human existence. A weakness or blockage of any one of these negatively affects the others and prevents their correct function. This always results in pathology of some kind. Tui Na skills brought to bear on meridians and their qi-points can strengthen these energetic substances and remove stagnation. Good health is an indication that they are all strong and in harmonious balance.

QI In TCM, the most fundamental of the energies is qi, because without qi nothing can happen. Qi causes change, movement, warmth, transformation and stability. Qi is really the same as the chemical energy of Western medicine and has the same origins. Qi is the vital life energy responsible for all living processes in nature.

Every new life requires qi to get started. It comes from the parents through the egg and sperm and is called 'yuan qi'. This is the one and only dose of inherited qi or original qi that the body receives. The **kidney** governs the body's reserves of yuan qi.

The qi needed throughout an individual's lifetime is produced from food and drink ('gu qi') by the **spleen** and from air ('kong qi') by the **lung**. This qi is called 'acquired qi'. There is nothing mysterious or magical about qi. It's the body's vital energy, which can manifest itself in many different ways. Qi enables us to grow, repair ourselves, reproduce, fight disease, maintain the body in a state of balance and carry us through from conception to the moment of death.

JING The second energy, jing, is a fundamental energetic 'substance'. It's like the energy of DNA, which you inherit from your parents. The **kidney** governs the body's reserves of jing.

Every person starts life with an equal injection of DNA from their mother and father. It comes through the egg and sperm. This is the source of inherited or original jing. After this one and only injection of inherited jing, the embryo has to make all its jing for the rest of its life.

This jing is acquired jing and, like qi, it comes from food, drink and air. It's important to have a good and well-balanced diet to ensure that you get all the chemicals in the right quantities to make the acquired jing and qi necessary for your body.

So we now have the two most vital ingredients for ensuring the correct functioning of the human body – qi, to make things happen; and jing, to control how, when and where they happen.

SHEN The third energetic 'substance' is shen. It's a manifestation of qi, responsible for the functioning of the mind and spirit. Shen is associated with a sparkling personality and plenty of vitality. It underpins consciousness, intelligence, memory, compassion and caring. Shen is controlled by jing and qi through the **heart**.

THE MATERIAL SUBSTANCES

Blood and body fluids are material substances that fundamentally affect the energetic functions of qi, jing and shen. By their physical nature, they are amenable to the effects of Tui Na, which can successfully remove blockages and strengthen their functions.

BLOOD The Chinese concept of blood has a wider meaning than 'blood' in Western medicine. It's also the energetic fluid of the body. Qi powers blood production from materials obtained from food and air, but qi in turn is nourished by blood. Qi and blood support each other to the extent that one cannot function without its partner.

BODY FLUIDS All the other natural body liquids, such as sweat, saliva, mucus, tears and joint fluid, are classified as 'body fluids'. Their function is to moisten the body tissues, muscles, organs, skin and hair and transport nutrients and qi from the blood to the tissues. Stagnated body fluids are called 'phlegm'. The lighter, clearer fluids, such as sweat and tears, are the 'jin', while the heavier, thicker fluids that lubricate the joints and provide cerebrospinal fluid are called 'ye'.

HOW CAN TUI NA AFFECT THE FIVE SUBSTANCES AND ORGAN FUNCTIONS?

Tui Na techniques should be applied to all meridians and to specific acupoints (see page 24) to stimulate functions of the five substances and remove stagnation. This in turn strengthens all the TCM organs.

COMPARISON BASED ON YIN AND YANG

YIN	YANG
ICE	WATER
WATER	STEAM
MIDNIGHT	MIDDAY
QUIET	LOUD
SLOW	FAST
COLD	HOT
INTERNAL	EXTERNAL
CHRONIC	ACUTE
DEFICIENCY	EXCESS

Yin and yang – the concept of relativity

The yin/yang symbol at the beginning of this chapter is a pictorial representation of the relativity that exists between yin and yang functions. All life processes involve the complex interaction of a vast number of different functions to achieve perfect balance. Some are labelled as 'yin' and some are 'yang'. They can be thought of as opposite ends of a spectrum. Yin functions are constantly interacting with yang ones, and through this interaction the right balance for every process is achieved. What is the right balance now may not be the right balance later because life processes are dynamic and ever-changing.

Every process has its yin and yang components. Yin and yang are only labels to define the relativeness of these components. Yin functions tend to be the less dynamic ones, while yang functions are forcefully dynamic. The ancient Chinese saw yin and yang as the shady and bright sides of the mountain, respectively. Nothing is absolutely yin or yang. Water, for example, is yin compared with steam but yang compared with ice. Midday is relatively more yang compared to midnight.

YIN AND YANG MERIDIAN BALANCE

All healthy physical, mental and spiritual processes are subject to balance between yin and yang. It's this

DAY

MIDDAY
relatively most yang and least yin

MIDNIGHT
relatively most yin and least yang

NIGHT

correct balance that determines good health. Any disturbance in the yin/yang relationship results in pathology of some kind.

ACUTE AND CHRONIC CONDITIONS

- Chronic conditions are deficiencies that develop over a period of time and indicate a weakness in the body's energies lasting months, years or, at worst, a lifetime.
- Acute conditions are excess. They develop rapidly and can be of short duration.
- An acute condition that does not clear up can develop into a chronic problem.

TUI NA DIAGNOSIS Careful palpation helps you to pinpoint painful areas on the yin and yang meridians and their qi-points. Together with knowledge of the five substances, organ functions and five elements, you will be able to devise an effective Tui Na treatment with focus on appropriate qi-points. Pain is the signal to show that qi is not flowing smoothly. Tui Na is the means of improving qi-flow.

TCM reasons for the origins of disease

Traditional Chinese medicine regards any disturbance to the body's health as originating from either the external climatic environment, from within the body itself or from injuries of all kinds, including surgery and unforeseen events.

EXTERNAL ORIGINS OF DISEASE

Many diseases originate from the exterior and are caused by climatic factors such as:
- wind
- cold
- damp
- heat
- dryness

The early Chinese knew nothing of bacteria or viruses. If the body's qi is strong, the invasion by pathogens will be easily repelled. If the body's qi function is weak, pathogens will invade and cause illness.

INTERNAL ORIGINS OF DISEASE

The most common internal origins of disturbed health are excessive and unresolved emotions. Any emotional

ORGAN	EMOTION
Liver	Anger, frustration, stress
Heart	Joy, anxiety
Spleen	Worry, overthinking
Lung	Grief, sadness
	Fear, panic

Organs and their associated emotions

state that is given no outlet can cause disease. Frequent bouts of excessive emotion are always harmful to health. They affect the functioning of the TCM internal organs, which are each related to specific emotions.

OTHER REASONS FOR DISEASE
- Poor diet, irregular eating habits, overeating and excessive dieting
- Excessive consumption of alcohol, smoking and the taking of recreational drugs
- Long-term use of Western medications and chemotherapy
- Excessive sex
- Overworking
- Sedentary lifestyle
- Too little or too much exercise
- Inadequate sleep

WHAT CAN TUI NA DO?

Regular Tui Na will help to maintain the improvements in your health brought about by lifestyle changes (see chapter 6, page 136). Tui Na applied skilfully to the meridians and their qi-points, with a clear understanding of the underlying theory, will strengthen all deficiencies and remove stagnation of qi and blood.

The TCM organs

In TCM, the organs are functional ones and do not correspond exactly to the physical organs of the same name in Western physiology. There is some overlap with the Western physiological functions, but, in addition, the organs in TCM have a different and much wider range of functions than corresponding Western organs. Not only do they control physical processes, but also the mind and emotions.

THE ZANG-FU In TCM the principal organs are the 'zang-fu'. The 'zang' organs are the lung, heart, pericardium, liver, spleen and kidney, which are all classified as yin, relative to the more yang 'fu' organs, the large intestine, small intestine, sanjiao, gall bladder, stomach and bladder.

Each organ is connected to the meridian that bears its name. Links between meridians provide for energetic connections between the organs. Each yin organ is

ZANG YIN ORGANS	FU YANG ORGANS
Lung – LU	Large Intestine – LI
Pericardium – P	Sanjiao – SJ
Heart – H	Small Intestine – SI
Spleen – SP	Stomach – ST
Liver – LIV	Gall Bladder – GB
Kidney – K	Bladder – BL

Organs and their abbreviations

linked with a yang organ to create a system where there is the potential for yin/yang functional balance.

For health, the organs must work together in harmony to sustain the body's activities. Qi, jing, shen, blood and body fluids must all function effectively to maintain the best yin/yang balance between the organs.

The principal functions of each of the organs are described with each meridian in chapter 3. The **five colours** refer to the **Five Elements** classification described on pages 20–21.

PERICARDIUM The pericardium (in Western medicine, the membrane surrounding the heart) is sometimes called the 'heart protector'. It's usually regarded as functioning as an extension to the heart organ energies.

SANJIAO The sanjiao has no equivalent in Western anatomy. In Chinese, it means 'three jiao' – the upper, middle and lower parts of the trunk, which contain the zang-fu organs. The function of the sanjiao is to regulate those organs. It's sometimes called the 'triple warmer' or 'triple burner'.

The meridians

The Chinese have long recognized that it's not only the quality of qi that is significant in maintaining health but the way it's distributed and balanced throughout the body. Every one of the billions of cells that make up the human body requires to be constantly suffused with qi and blood to enable it to live and function normally. In TCM, the meridians perform this essential function.

The meridians are not physical channels in the way that veins and arteries are channels for blood. They cannot be examined by dissection. The meridian system has been well documented in Chinese medicine for more than 2,000 years, and it has recently been confirmed by scientific experiments, which show that the meridians have unique and different electrical potentials from the surrounding tissues. The meridians are electrically charged energetic pathways through the body's tissues, along which qi currents flow. Their precise routes have been traced and found to correspond to those on ancient Chinese meridian charts and Chinese bronzes. The flow of qi in the meridians can be likened to the world's great ocean currents, which follow clearly defined routes through the seas.

THE TWELVE PRIMARY MERIDIANS LAYOUT

Each meridian has a qi-flow linked with one of the principal internal organs after which it's named. There are twelve organ-linked meridians. Each meridian is represented equally and symmetrically in both halves of the body. Six of the meridians are labelled as yin because they are linked with the six organs that have a more yin function. The other six are described as yang because they are linked to the more yang organs.

YIN MERIDIANS	YANG MERIDIANS
Lung – LU	Large Intestine – LI
Pericardium – P	Sanjiao – SJ
Heart – H	Small Intestine – SI
Spleen – SP	Stomach – ST
Liver – LIV	Gall Bladder – GB
Kidney – K	Bladder – BL

Twelve main meridians and their abbreviations, using five colours to represent the Five Elements described on pages 20–21.

THE FIVE ELEMENTS

Early Chinese philosophy recognized five energies that dominate the universe, including all life processes. They called them the Five Elements: fire, water, earth, wood and metal. In this way of thinking about the nature of existence, the human body and mind are also subject to the energies of these elements. Each zang-fu organ pair and its associated meridians is influenced by one of the five elemental energies. Each meridian pair is classified according to this Five Element relationship and colour-coded according to the colour associated with each element (see opposite).

Any imbalances in the energies of one element will show up as symptoms in one or both of the organs in the pair and in their meridians. For example, an imbalance in the wood element can affect the liver or gall bladder organs and meridians, or both. The associations between the organs, their meridians and the elements are shown in the outer ring of the diagram on the facing page. Each element (in the inner ring of the diagram) dominates one organ pair (on the outer ring), with the exception of fire, which influences two pairs: the heart and small intestine, and the pericardium and sanjiao.

The diagram also shows the relationship between the elements and other 'correspondences'. Each element has a related emotion, and also a specific body part. For example, bones are related to water, and bone problems such as osteoarthritis could reflect an imbalance in the water element.

It is the same for the relevant outlet in the body. The ear is the outlet related to water, and any imbalance of water energies could affect the sense of hearing. Each element is also linked with a particular season, a type of weather and a taste, all of which are shown in the diagram.

This network of elemental associations reflects the complex ways that we interact with our environment and provides a way of describing and explaining the effects of this interaction. A knowledge of the Five Element theory can assist a Chinese medical

practitioner in interpreting a patient's emotional and physical state and in making a diagnosis.

The Five Elements also interact with each other in the same way that they do in nature. Wood produces fire (as fuel), fire produces earth (as ashes), earth produces metal (as ore), metal produces water (molten metal is liquid) and water produces wood (by feeding trees). This cycle is indicated by the clockwise arrows in the centre of the diagram on the facing page. In the same way, the organs corresponding to the Five Elements are linked in a creative cycle, with each element passing energy on to the next. In this way the liver (wood) sustains and supports the heart (fire), which in turn supports the spleen (earth).

An untreated problem in the organs associated with wood, for example, could lead to imbalance in fire, resulting in insomnia. If the fire energy is low, with the patient being weak and pale, the wood energies need strengthening

There is also a control cycle, shown by the second set of arrows in the centre of the diagram, which similarly reflects interactions in nature. For example, in the body, a heart excess condition such as insomnia and a red face can be controlled by the water element. Water controls fire by extinguishing it, so strengthening the kidney can treat insomnia.

The symbols inside the diagram, opposite, represent the Five Elements. Starting at the top, and following the clockwise arrows, they are: fire, earth, metal, water and wood. The set of arrows at the centre of the diagram indicate the elements that can interact with each other to treat different conditions.

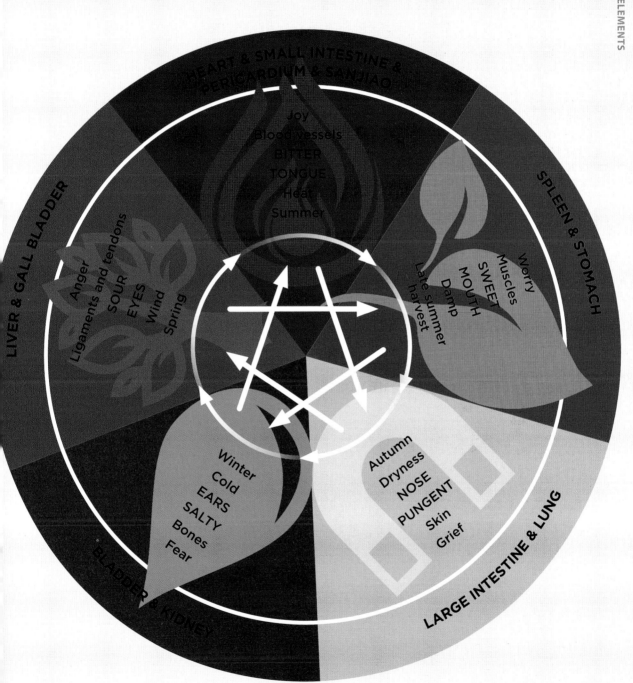

HEART & SMALL INTESTINE & PERICARDIUM & SANJIAO

Joy
Blood vessels
BITTER
TONGUE
Heat
Summer

SPLEEN & STOMACH

Worry
Muscles
SWEET
MOUTH
Damp
Late summer
harvest

LIVER & GALL BLADDER

Anger
Ligaments and tendons
SOUR
EYES
Wind
Spring

Winter
Cold
EARS
SALTY
Bones
Fear

Autumn
Dryness
NOSE
PUNGENT
Skin
Grief

LARGE INTESTINE & LUNG

BLADDER & KIDNEY

MERIDIANS AND QI-POINTS

• • • • • • • • • • • • • • • • • • •

The classical system of meridians and their qi-points was first mapped, and was already well established, more than 2,000 years ago. On these meridians there are more than 360 qi-points where qi can be affected in a way that restores balance and harmony.

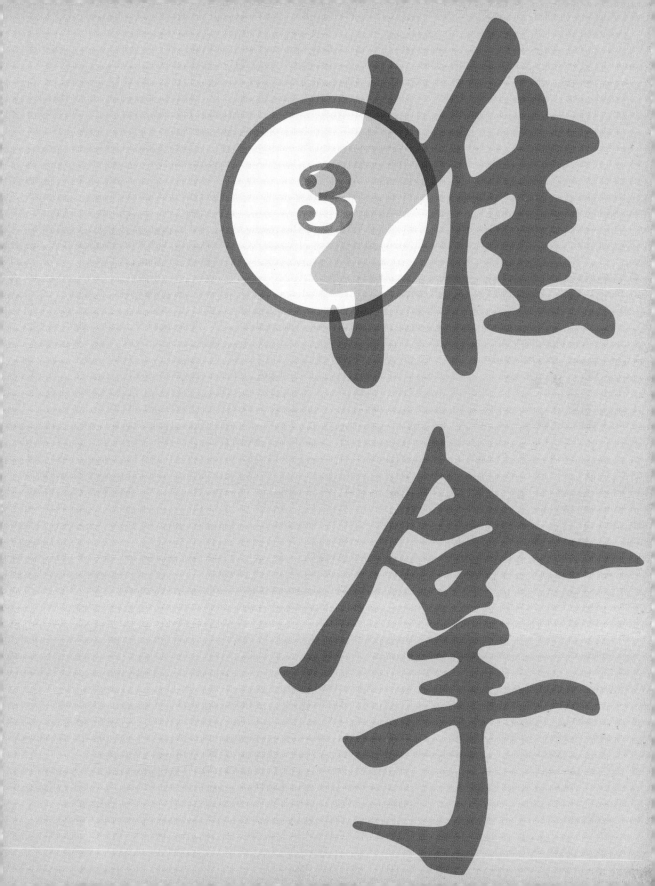

3 雅拿

Qi-points

At various intervals along the meridians there are specific points, each with its own unique electrical potential. Acupuncturists call them 'acupoints', but in this Tui Na book they are called 'qi-points'.

In Tui Na, these points can be stimulated by strong pressure, or by needling or cupping. Each qi-point has the potential to affect qi and blood flow in the local tissues but also throughout its meridian, its associated organ and in related meridians. Such is the power of Tui Na that all qi-points are uniquely able to strengthen qi and blood flow as well as remove blockages that cause stagnation.

In the West, the qi-points are all numbered and named according to the meridian on which they are found – for example, Gall Bladder 20 or Large Intestine 4. The standard abbreviations for these are given in the table on page 19. I have chosen qi-points that are particularly powerful and effective in Tui Na, and are most useful for maintaining health, relieving muscle and joint pain and treating many common health problems.

A Tui Na practitioner questions the patient about symptoms and location of pain or discomfort and palpates painful areas to discover which meridian or meridians are primarily affected. From this, and knowledge of meridians and qi-points, the practitioner decides the specific meridians on which to apply Tui Na massage techniques and the specific qi-points on which to focus. For a more comprehensive diagnosis, it would be necessary to identify patterns of disharmony involving the 'five substances', the organs and their yin/yang status (see page 16).

Every qi-point has clearly defined therapeutic functions. Kneading or pressing repetitively on a qi-point will affect qi-flow in a specific way unique to that particular qi-point. The author believes that it's necessary to knead the chosen points with at least one hundred repetitions where a particular problem has to be resolved, or fifty repetitions for general healthcare.

FINDING QI-POINTS

The positions of qi-points are given with reference to body landmarks. The 'cun' (pronounced 'soon') is a non-standard unit, used in Chinese medicine to measure the distance of qi-points from body landmarks, such as bones and muscles.

A cun varies from person to person (see diagram opposite). Distances between parts of the body, however, have fixed cun measurements regardless

of the size of the body (see Appendix, page 153). For example, the distance from the lateral knee to the lateral ankle is always 16 cun, while the distance from elbow crease to wrist crease is 12 cun. The meridian illustrations on pages 32–59 show the qi-points and describe their positions using this system. Practise finding qi-points, both on yourself and your partner, so that you are familiar with the measuring technique before you start on the whole-body routine in chapter 5. A qi-point that feels particularly tender or even painful to the touch may indicate an underlying energy or musculoskeletal problem in the meridian that needs focused kneading to correct qi-flow.

THE CUN MEASUREMENT A single cun is the width of the top of your own thumb, not the thumb of the therapist. The combined width of the index and middle finger is 1.5 cun; and the four fingers together make 3 cun. As the cun varies from one person to another, you need to use the width of your partner's own fingers to give you their cun measurement in order to locate their qi-points accurately.

USING QI-POINTS AND ASHI POINTS

Where qi-points are recommended for healthcare or treatment for common ailments, you should knead them bilaterally – that is, on both sides of the body – to boost qi and blood circulation and remove stagnation. The twelve paired meridians occur symmetrically on either side of the body.

Sometimes during a massage painful points are found that do not lie directly on a meridian. Such points are called 'ashi points' or 'painful points'. When treating a local pain or injury, use the local qi-points on the side affected and nearby ashi points to get the best results.

For clarity, the qi-points are illustrated on only one side of the body, and each point is labelled on the illustration with the meridian abbreviation. Captions give the Western qi-point numbers and their Chinese names (see below), clear instructions for finding the qi-points and a list of conditions that they treat.

CHINESE NAMES The Chinese use specific names and not the Western numbering system to describe the qi-points. The names reflect either the position or the function of the point.

YINXIANG – LI 20 This translates as 'welcome fragrance' or 'meeting of a good smell'. Found in the depression on

MEASURING CUN

See Appendix, page 153,
for fixed cun measurements.

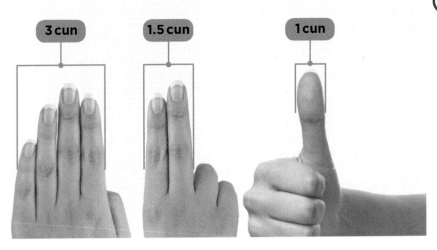

3 cun   1.5 cun   1 cun

the outside of the nostril, it is the final point of the large intestine meridian. Massage on **LI 20** helps to clear a blocked nose, enabling it to smell fragrant scents again – hence the name 'welcome fragrance'.

YUJI – LU 10 The point, meaning 'fish belly', is at the base of the thumb, where the skin changes colour and type. The name refers to the large muscle at the base of the thumb, which resembles a fish belly.

TIANZHU – BL 10 The point, which is on the neck, translates as 'celestial pillar' or 'column of heaven' and represents the pillar that supports the head.

JINGMENG – BL 1 Meaning 'eye brightness', this point at the inner corner of the eye is used for treating eye disorders, thus brightening the eyes.

ZUSANLI – ST 36 This point, meaning 'walk three miles', is 3 cun (see above) below the lateral knee 'eye' and 1 cun outside the crest of the tibia. It strengthens the whole body's qi and stamina, enabling you to walk with no effort.

PISHU – BL 20 Located 1.5 cun from the spinous process (a bony projection) of the eleventh thoracic vertebra, the point is named 'pishu' ('spleen point') because it tonifies all the functions of the spleen organ.

LOCAL AND DISTAL QI-POINTS It's worth having a knowledge of the muscles and joints through which the meridians pass because local qi-points can be used to treat musculoskeletal problems in their immediate vicinity. These can be reinforced with selected distal qi-points on the same meridian. With joint or muscle pain it's essential to palpate to find the painful qi-points or ashi points and knead them for several minutes. As a beginner, it may be difficult to pinpoint exactly the site

of the pain. Identify the meridians that pass through the painful area and use Tui Na techniques to thoroughly massage along them.

Examples of local qi-points

- **SI 11** on the scapula treats shoulder blade pain.
- **SJ 14** on the deltoid muscle treats posterior shoulder pain and immobility.
- **BL 23** on the lumbar region strengthens kidney function and treats lower back pain.
- **ST 7** treats toothache in the lower jaw.

Examples of distal qi-points

Qi-points on the lower limbs are called distal points. These are used for problems in other parts of the body, frequently on the same meridian. Distal qi-points are also useful for treating conditions where local points cannot be used because of skin problems or severe bruising.

- **SI 3** on the hand treats shoulder blade pain.
- **SJ 5** just above the wrist treats posterior shoulder pain and immobility.
- **BL 60** treats lower back pain.
- **ST 44** on the foot treats toothache.

When you are familiar with the exact routes of the twelve primary meridians, you can start thinking about their yin and yang relationships, which you can utilize in your treatments. A diagnosis of the patient will indicate which of the organs and fundamental substances need treatment. The focus of the Tui Na massage should be on the meridians and qi-points related to these organs. Qi-points that need specific attention are often the ones that feel tender or painful when palpated.

Tui Na is thus a very precise therapy. The whole-body routine set out in chapter 5 involves working along meridians and kneading qi-points. To give a successful Tui Na massage, you should know the route and direction of every meridian and where it starts and ends. Learning the exact anatomical positions and functions of each qi-point described in this book will ensure that you achieve excellent results. This will enable you to focus specifically on a wide range of conditions.

BACK SHU QI-POINTS

In addition to their specific, therapeutic, local functions, qi-points on the part of the bladder meridian that runs from the neck to the sacrum, down either side of the spine, are called 'back shu'. They are used to treat local back pain, but each qi-point has a specific link to one of the zang-fu organs after which it's named. For example, while kneading **BL 21**, the stomach shu point has a powerful effect on stomach

functions. Three of the qi-points – **BL 11**, **BL 12** and **BL 17** – on this part of the meridian are not 'shu' points but 'influential points'.

For a quick and effective treatment to maintain good health, a Tui Na massage covering all the back shu points will stimulate all the body's organs, boosting and balancing qi-flow and removing any blockages. Work through all these points, as described in the back massage section, in Part Three of the whole-body routine in chapter 5.

FRONT MU QI-POINTS

On the chest and abdomen, there are qi-points that have special links with the organs and are known as 'mu' qi-points. For example, while kneading **R 12**, the stomach mu point has a powerful effect on stomach function.

OUTER BLADDER POINTS	BACK SHU POINTS	RELATED ORGANS	FRONT MU POINTS
BL 42	BL 13	Lung	LU 1
BL 43	BL 14	Pericardium	R 17
BL 44	BL 15	Heart	R 14
BL 47	BL 18	Liver	LIV 14
BL 48	BL 19	Gall Bladder	GB 24
BL 49	BL 20	Spleen	LIV 13
BL 50	BL 21	Stomach	R 12
BL 51	BL 22	Sanjiao	R 5
BL 52	BL 23	Kidney	GB 25
	BL 25	Large Intestine	ST 25
	BL 27	Small Intestine	R 4
	BL 28	Bladder	R 3

OUTER BLADDER POINTS	INFLUENTIAL POINTS	
	BL 11	Bone
BL 41	BL 12	Wind
BL 46	BL 17	Blood/Diaphragm

The principal functions of each of the organs are described with each meridian in chapter 3, page 32 onwards. The colours refer to the Five Elements described on pages 20–21. The outer bladder back points are level with the back shu points and have similar functions.

The energetic links between the twelve meridians

The simplest way of classifying meridians is according to their yin/yang relationships (see pages 17–19). In yin meridians the qi-flow is in the opposite direction to that in their yang partners, forming a continuous qi circuit. These partners connect through branches called collaterals. This energetic connection between the yin and yang meridians means that you could massage the yin meridian and knead qi-points on it to influence functions of the yang meridian, and vice versa. Massaging the meridians will in turn affect the associated organ functions.

LOCATION OF THE HAND AND FOOT MERIDIANS

TCM theory classifies the twelve meridians based on their relative yin-ness and yang-ness. The ancient Chinese tried to explain yin and yang by observing the sun shining on a mountain. The bright side is more yang and the shady side is relatively more yin. The yin meridians are located on the less exposed surfaces, and the yang meridians can be found on the more exposed surfaces.

Each meridian pair is dominated by the energies of one of the Five Elements (see pages 20–21), and the pages that follow present the meridians according to their ruling element. They describe the functions of the organs and meridians associated with each element, and the qi-points for treating problems that result from their functional imbalance.

These pages are coded using the colours associated with the elements: red for fire, green for wood, and so on. Illustrations of the meridians show all the qi-points used in the treatments in chapters 5 and 6.

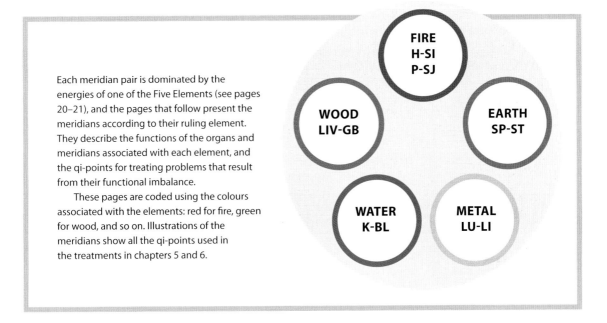

FIRE
H-SI
P-SJ

WOOD
LIV-GB

EARTH
SP-ST

WATER
K-BL

METAL
LU-LI

Qi-flow of the yin/yang hand meridians

The flow of qi through the meridians of the hand link each hand yin meridian (lung, pericardium, heart) energetically with its hand yang meridian partners (large intestine, sanjiao, small intestine). You can trace the flow of qi through the six yin/yang hand meridians.

They are called hand meridians because they either start on the hand or end on the hand. The yin hand meridians start on the chest and end on the hand, whereas the yang hand meridians start on the hand and end on the head.

EXAMPLE: Starting with the lung yin meridian, the energy flows from the chest at LU 1 **down to the thumb**, and connects via collaterals to the large intestine yang meridian, which starts on the index finger LI 1 and **flows up to the face**, ending at LI 20.

You can trace the same circuits with the pericardium/sanjiao and heart/small intestine meridians. When you have learned the Tui Na techniques, you can use them to promote stronger qi-flow through these circuits, which in turn will promote health.

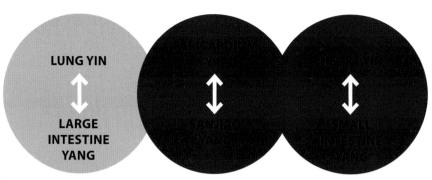

EXAMPLES

- Massaging along the **lung** yin meridian, focusing on LU 1, LU 5, LU 7 and LU 10, can prevent and treat colds due to weak lung organ function. As there is an energetic link with its yang partner, the **large intestine** meridian, you can reinforce this effect by kneading qi-points such as LI 4 and LI 11. See meridian points on pages 50–51.

- Anterior shoulder and elbow pain can be treated by massaging along the **large intestine** yang meridian, focusing on LI 15. As there is an energetic link with its yin partner, the **lung** meridian, you can reinforce its effect by kneading qi-points such as LU1 and LU 2.

Qi-flow of the yin/yang foot meridians

The qi-flow through the foot meridians links each foot **yin** meridian energetically with its foot **yang** meridian partner. As with the hand meridians, you can trace the flow of qi through the six yin/yang foot meridians. They are called foot meridians because they either start on the foot or end on the foot. The yin foot meridians start on the foot and end on the chest, while the yang foot meridians start on the head and end on the feet.

EXAMPLE: Starting with the spleen yin meridian, the energy flows from the big toe at SP 1 **up to the chest**, connects via collaterals to the stomach yang meridian, which starts just under the eye at ST 1, and flows **down to the foot**, ending at ST 45 on the second toe.

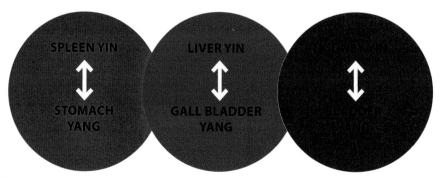

EXAMPLES

- To treat headaches, which are often caused by qi stagnation, massage the **gall bladder** yang meridian, focusing on qi-points such as GB 20, GB 21, GB 8 and GB 14. Intensify their effect by massaging qi-points LIV 3, LIV 8 and LIV 13 on its yin partner, the **liver** meridian.

- To treat medial knee pain, massage the **liver** yin meridian, focusing on qi-point LIV 8. To intensify the effect, massage qi-point GB 34 on its yang partner, the **gall bladder** meridian. See meridian points on pages 32–5.

Eight extraordinary meridians

In addition, there are eight 'extraordinary' meridians, only two of which are described here. They are the **ren** and **du** meridians, which encircle the head and trunk on the midline. In English, the ren meridian is called the 'conception vessel' and du is called the 'governing vessel'. The ren meridian is relatively more yin than the more yang du meridian.
(See also pages 58–9.)

FUNCTIONS OF THE REN YIN AND DU YANG MERIDIANS

NOTE: Problems on these meridians should be treated with Tui Na massage applied along them, with focused kneading of appropriate qi-points.

THE REN YIN MERIDIAN

This regulates the six hand/foot yin meridians. The three yin meridians of the foot cross at R3 and R4.

Recommended qi-points for treatment
- Kidney, spleen and liver dysfunction **R 4**
- Bladder dysfunction **R 3**
- Stomach and spleen dysfunction **R 12, R 10**
- Heart dysfunction **R 14, R 17**
- Lung dysfunction **R 17, R 22**
- Qi deficiency **R 6, R 12**
- Blood deficie ncy **R 4**
- Reproductive problems **R 3, R 4**

THE DU YANG MERIDIAN

This regulates six hand/foot yang meridians. They cross at DU 14 and DU 20.

Recommended qi-points for treatment
- Kidney dysfunction **DU 4**
- Lower back pain **DU 3, DU 4**
- Qi and yang deficiency **DU 14**
- Depression and emotional stress **DU 20**
- Resuscitation point **DU 26**

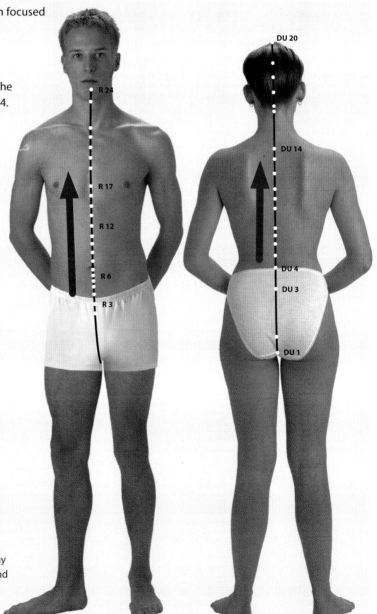

The **ren meridian** starts midway between the anus and the genitals, and the **du meridian** starts midway between the tip of the coccyx and the anus. They end just below and above the mouth, respectively.

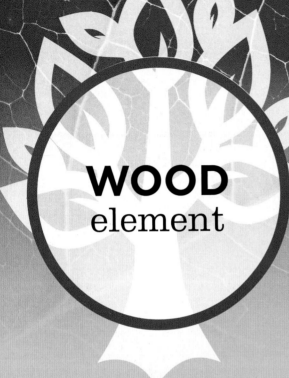

WOOD
element

The **liver yin** and the **gall bladder yang** are the **foot** yin/yang meridian partners and are each energetically linked to their named organ. Both are classified under the **wood element** in the Five Elements.

FUNCTIONS OF THE LIVER YIN ORGAN

REGULATES THE DISTRIBUTION OF QI AND BLOOD FUNCTION Weak liver qi function affects the smooth and unobstructed access of qi and blood to all the organs. It can cause menstrual problems, oedema and pain anywhere along the meridian, such as pain in the breasts and under the lower ribs.

REGULATES DIGESTION If liver qi function is disturbed, all kinds of digestive problems can arise, including bloating, nausea and vomiting.

REGULATES ALL EMOTIONAL ACTIVITIES Sudden, extreme emotions will disturb the liver function.

STORES BLOOD Weak liver function can cause dizziness, weak limbs and muscle spasms, scanty or profuse menstruation and high blood pressure.

CONTROLS THE HEALTHY FUNCTION OF TENDONS Malfunction of the liver can result in stiff joints and difficulty bending and stretching.

LIVER YIN (LIV) AND GALL BLADDER YANG (GB)

THE LIVER YIN MERIDIAN
Recommended qi-points for treatment:

- headaches, dizziness **LIV 3, LIV 2**
- PMT with abdominal pain **LIV 3, LIV 8, LIV 13, LIV 14**
- impotence, genital pain and itching **LIV 5**
- indigestion **LIV 13**
- medial knee pain **LIV 8, LIV 7**
- medial ankle pain **LIV 4**
- anger **LIV 3, LIV 2**

THE GALL BLADDER YANG MERIDIAN
Recommended qi-points for treatment:

- migraine **GB 8, GB 14, GB 20, GB 21, GB 43, GB 44**
- ear problems **GB 2, GB 12, GB 43**
- pain around the ribs **GB 34, GB 24**
- neck pain **GB 20, GB 12**
- shoulder pain **GB 21**
- side lumbar pain **GB 25**
- hip pain **GB 30, GB 29**
- side of leg pain **GB 31, GB 34**
- knee pain **GB 34**
- outer ankle pain **GB 40, GB 39**
- sore, red or achy eyes **GB 1, GB 20, GB14, GB 43**
- emotional upset **GB 13**

NOTE: problems on these meridians should be treated with Tui Na massage applied along them, with focused kneading of appropriate qi-points and related back shu points BL 18 and BL 19 and front mu points LIV 14 and GB 24.

IS REFLECTED IN THE CONDITION OF THE NAILS Impaired liver function causes pale, brittle, dry or ridged nails.

HAS ITS CONNECTION WITH THE EXTERIOR THROUGH THE EYES Disturbed liver function results in blurred vision, night blindness, and itchy and red eyes.

IS LINKED TO THE ANGER EMOTION Uncontrolled liver qi can cause frustration, depression and severe stress.

FUNCTIONS OF THE GALL BLADDER YANG ORGAN
RECEIVES, STORES AND DISCHARGES BILE As yin/yang partners, the liver and gall bladder strongly interact. Weak gall bladder function causes poor digestion, hypochondriac pain and vomiting.

LIVER
yin
meridian

LIV 1 is on the inner margin of the big toe just behind the nail, and the meridian ends at **LIV 14**, between the sixth and seventh ribs directly below the nipple. Opposite are the main Tui Na qi-points, listed from top to bottom. For **front mu** points, see page 26.

LIV 14 QIMEN Liver front mu
Below the nipple in the space between the sixth and seventh ribs. *It removes stagnation and improves qi-flow; reduces lumps in the breast and eases local chest pain.*

LIV 13 ZHANGMEN Spleen front mu
Directly in front of and just below the end of the eleventh rib. *It improves interaction between liver and spleen for efficient digestion; tonifies all yin organs.*

LIV 8 QUQUAN
On the inner side of the leg, just above the knee crease between two big tendons. *Tones the hamstring muscles; treats knee pain.*

LIV 7 XIGUAN
Slide up the inside edge of the tibia to where the bone flares – this is SP 9. LIV 7 is 1 cun behind SP 9. *Treats medial knee pain.*

LIV 5 LIGOU
5 cun above the inner ankle bone, just off the edge of the tibia. *Treats impotence, and pain and itching in the genitals.*

LIV 4 ZHONGFENG
In a depression anterior to the head of the medial maleolus. *Treats ankle and foot pain.*

LIV 3 TAICHONG
In a depression just in front of the point where the first and second metatarsal bones come together. *Improves qi-flow and calms emotions; treats headaches, menstruation problems and PMT, and improves eye health.*

LIV 2 XINGJIAN
Between the first and second toes, 0.5 cun behind the web. *Treats headache, inflamed red eyes, irritability, anger, menstruation problems and numb toes.*

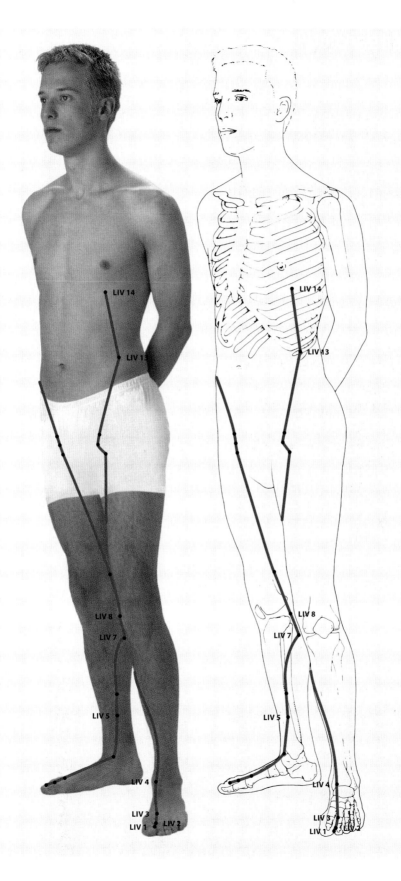

LIV 14

LIV 13

LIV 14

LIV 13

LIV 8
LIV 7

LIV 8
LIV 7

LIV 5

LIV 5

LIV 4

LIV 4

LIV 3
LIV 1   LIV 2

LIV 3
LIV 1   LIV 2

GALL BLADDER
yang meridian

This meridian starts at **GB 1**, in a small depression at the outer corner of the eye, and ends at **GB 44** on the outer margin of the fourth toe just behind the nail. Opposite are the main Tui Na qi-points, listed from top to bottom. For **front mu** points, see page 26.

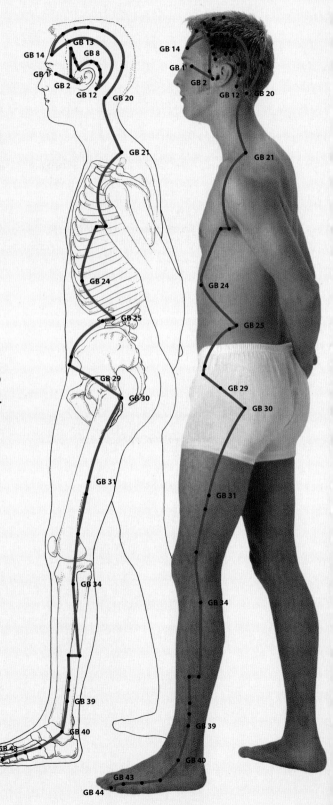

GB 14 GB 13 GB 8 GB 14
GB 1 GB 1
GB 2 GB 2
GB 12 GB 20 GB 12 GB 20
GB 21 GB 21
GB 24 GB 24
GB 25 GB 25
GB 29 GB 29
GB 30 GB 30
GB 31 GB 31
GB 34 GB 34
GB 39 GB 39
GB 40 GB 40
GB 43 GB 43
GB 44 GB 44

GB 1 TONGZILIAO
In a depression at the outer corner of the eye. *Maintains healthy eyes and treats soreness, redness and twitching.*

GB 2 TINGHUI
In a depression felt when the mouth is open, just in front of the ear, level with the lower border of the tragus. *Benefits hearing and treats tinnitus.*

GB 8 SHUAIGU
1.5 cun directly above the top of the ear. *Treats migraine headaches.*

GB 12 WANGU
Behind and below the mastoid process of the skull. *Treats headaches, neck tension and ear problems, and calms the mind for good sleep.*

GB 13 BENSHEN
3 cun from the midline of the forehead and 0.5 cun above the hairline. *Calms the mind, treats psychological problems.*

GB 14 YANGBAI
1 cun above the midpoint of the eyebrow. *Improves qi-flow to the eyes, forehead and brain; treats frontal headaches and twitching eyelids.*

GB 20 FENGCHI
At the top of the nape of the neck, in the depression immediately below the base of the skull. It prevents qi and blood stagnation in the brain, reducing the potential for strokes. *Treats all kinds of headaches, neck tension, problems affecting eyes and ears, flu and common cold, hypertension, Parkinson's syndrome and epilepsy.*

GB 21 JIANJING
In the middle of a line drawn from the spinous process of cervical vertebra seven to the edge of the shoulder joint (acromion). *Relaxes shoulder and neck muscles; treats shoulder pain and tension headaches.*

GB 24 RIYUE Gall bladder front mu
Below the nipple, in the space between the seventh and eight ribs. *Complements LIV 14, regulating liver and gall bladder qi.*

GB 25 JINGMEN Kidney front mu
On the outer lower back at the free end of the twelfth rib. *Strengthens and treats the lower back.*

GB 29 JULIAO
Halfway between the top and front of the iliac spine to the outer edge of the hip bone. *Treats side hip and leg pain.*

GB 30 HUANTIAO
One-third of the way along a line from the outer edge of the hip bone to the coccyx. *Relaxes the hip joint and buttock muscles; treats local pain and sciatica, and weakness and pain in the lower leg.*

GB 31 FENGSHI
On the side of the thigh, just less than halfway (7 cun) from the knee crease to the hip bone (19 cun). *Releases side leg tension and pain; treats sciatica.*

GB 34 YANGLINGQUAN
In the depression just in front of and slightly below the head of the fibula. Relaxes tendons, ligaments and muscle fascia throughout the body. *Treats sciatica and muscle spasm, weakness in the leg, and knee and ankle pain.*

GB 39 XUANZHONG
Just in front of the edge of the fibula, 3 cun above the tip of the outer ankle bone. *Strengthens 'marrow' to build up bones and boost brain function.*

GB 40 QIUXU
In a depression, at the lower front edge of the outer ankle bone. *Maintains ankle mobility; treats ankle sprain.*

GB 43 XIAXI
Between the fourth and fifth toes just above the web. *Improves blood flow to the toes; treats dizziness, headache, red and painful eyes.*

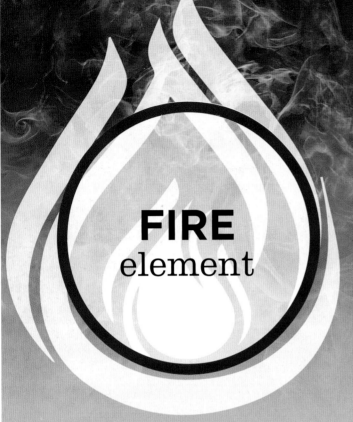

FIRE
element

Four meridians are classified under the **fire element** in Five Element theory. The **heart yin** and the **small intestine yang**, and the **pericardium yin** and the **sanjiao yang**, are the **hand** yin/yang meridian partners, which are each energetically linked to their named organs.

FUNCTIONS OF THE HEART YIN ORGAN

REGULATES BLOOD AND QI PRODUCTION Overworking or lack of sleep can deplete heart qi and blood to cause tiredness, breathlessness, pallor and palpitations.

POWERS BLOOD FLOW IN THE BLOOD VESSELS Heart qi maintains healthy blood pressure to prevent the onset of palpitations and cardiac pain.

COMPLEXION REFLECTS HEART FUNCTION Weak blood flow results in a purplish or bluish tinge to the lips, tongue and facial skin.

CONTROLS THE SHEN Impaired heart qi results in weak or disturbed shen, which can cause insomnia, dream-disturbed sleep and depression.

HAS ITS CONNECTION WITH THE EXTERIOR THROUGH THE TONGUE Disturbed heart qi can cause tongue ulcers, stiff tongue and speech defects.

LINKS TO THE JOY EMOTION Heart qi and blood malfunction can cause anxiety, joylessness and a tendency to get overexcited.

FUNCTIONS OF THE SMALL INTESTINE YANG ORGAN

CONTRIBUTES TO THE FORMATION OF BLOOD THROUGH DIGESTION
Abnormal absorption of fluids can result in constipation or loose stools and scanty or profuse urination.

FUNCTIONS OF THE PERICARDIUM YIN ORGAN

THE PERICARDIUM IS THE HEART PROTECTOR In TCM, the pericardium assists heart organ functions to strengthen the physical heart and balance the shen. Weak pericardium function often causes angina, palpitations and emotional agitation.

FUNCTIONS OF THE SANJIAO YANG ORGAN

REGULATES AND BALANCES QI BETWEEN THE THREE JIAO The sanjiao coordinates organ qi functions between the three jiao (see page 19). Sanjiao malfunction can disturb all the interactions between the lung, spleen and kidney.

HEART YIN (H), SMALL INTESTINE YANG (SI), PERICARDIUM YIN (P), SANJIAO HAND YANG (SJ) MERIDIANS

HEART YIN MERIDIAN
Recommended qi-points for treatment:

- heart problems, palpitations H 3, H 7, BL 15, R 14
- depression, heartbreak, panic, insomnia H 7, BL 15
- wrist pain H 7
- golfer's elbow H 3

PERICARDIUM YIN MERIDIAN
Recommended qi-points for treatment:

- vomiting and nausea P 6
- heart problems, angina, palpitations P 6, P 3, BL 14, R 17
- emotional upsets P 6, P7, P 8, R 17
- carpal tunnel syndrome P 7, P 6, P 8, P 3

SMALL INTESTINE YANG MERIDIAN
Recommended qi-points for treatment:

- shoulder blade pain SI 11, SI 12
- upper shoulder pain SI 13, SI 14, SI 15
- centre back and neck pain SI 3
- back of arm pain SI 9, SI 10
- ear pain or deafness SI 19
- painful urination R 3
- elbow pain SI 8

SANJIAO HAND YANG MERIDIAN
Recommended qi-points for treatment:

- ear problems SJ 17, SJ 21, SJ 3, SJ 5
- eye problems SJ 23
- migraine SJ 5
- neck pain SJ 3, SJ 5, SJ 15
- arm and shoulder joint pain SJ 14, SJ 15, SJ 5
- elbow pain SJ 10
- lower abdominal pain R 5 (contraindicated in pregnancy)

NOTE: problems on these hand meridians should be treated with Tui Na massage applied along them, with focused kneading of appropriate qi-points and related back shu points BL 15, BL 28, BL 14 and BL 22 and front mu points R14, R 3, R17 and R 5 energetically linked to their named organs.

HEART
yin meridian

H 1 is in the centre of the armpit, and the heart meridian ends at **H 9**, at the base of the little fingernail on the inside edge. Below are the main Tui Na qi-points, listed from top to bottom.

H 3 SHAOHAI
At the inner end of the crease formed when the arm is flexed at the elbow. *Reduces potential for repetitive strain injury in the elbow; treats local elbow pain, such as golfer's elbow, and cardiac pain.*

H 7 SHENMEN
On the underside of the wrist, in line with the little finger, in a depression on the main wrist crease. *Calms a restless mind for better sleep; treats insomnia, depression, cardiac pain, palpitations and tongue ulcers.*

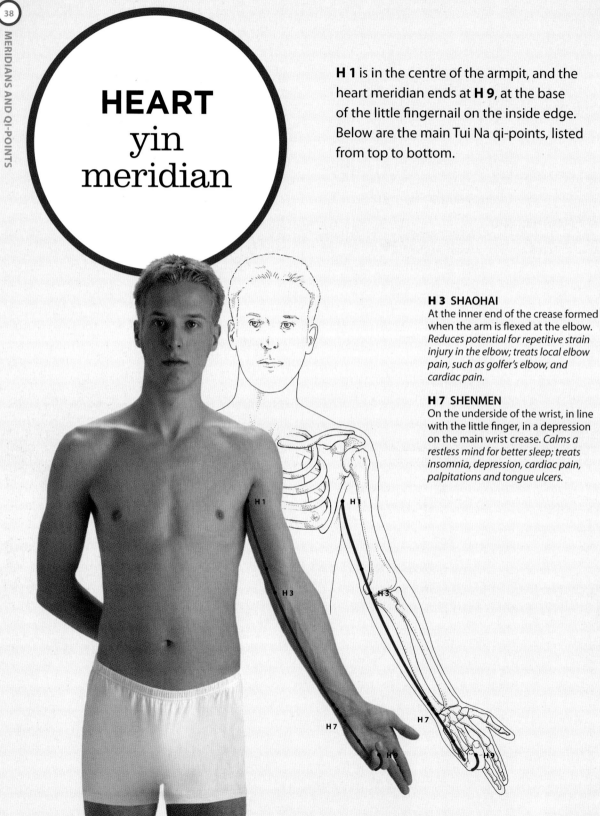

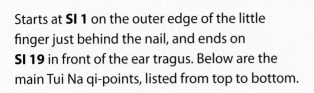

SMALL INTESTINE
yang meridian

Starts at **SI 1** on the outer edge of the little finger just behind the nail, and ends on **SI 19** in front of the ear tragus. Below are the main Tui Na qi-points, listed from top to bottom.

SI 19 TIANGGONG
In front of the ear tragus in a depression, when the mouth is open. *Promotes good hearing.*

SI 15 JIANZHONSHU
2 cun from the midline, level with the lower border of cervical vertebra seven. *Treats neck stiffness and pain.*

SI 14 JIANWAISHU
Just off the upper medial angle of the scapula, 3 cun from the midline, level with the lower border of thoracic vertebra one. *Treats pain and tension between the shoulder blades.*

SI 13 QUYUAN
On the top of the medial angle of the scapula, level with the lower border of the thoracic vertebra two. *Treats upper back stiffness and pain.*

SI 12 BINGFENG
Vertically up from SI 11 just over the scapular spine. *Treats upper shoulder and scapular pain.*

SI 11 TIANZONG
One-third of the way down the scapula. *Relaxes and treats pain in the scapular muscles.*

SI 10 NAOSHU
Above SI 9, below the outer end of the scapula. *Relaxes and treats pain in the shoulder.*

SI 9 JIANZHEN
1 cun above back armpit crease. *Relaxes and treats the shoulder muscles.*

SI 8 XIAOHAI
At the end of the olecranon process of the ulna. *Treats elbow pain.*

SI 3 HOUXI
On the outer end of the main crease formed by the knuckles of the clenched fist. *Treats local hand pain, and improves qi-flow to the spine to relieve neck and back pain.*

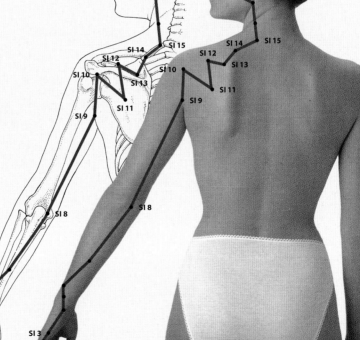

PERICARDIUM
yin meridian

P 1 is on the chest just beside the nipple in the space between the fourth and fifth ribs. The meridian ends at **P 9** on the centre of the tip of the middle finger. Below are the main Tui Na qi-points, listed from top to bottom.

P 3 QUZE
On the elbow crease just inside the tendon of the biceps muscle. *Maintains effective heart function to prevent cardiac pain and palpitations; treats golfer's elbow.*

P 6 NEIGUAN
On the underside of the forearm, 2 cun above the middle crease on the wrist, in the midline between the two large tendons. *Regular stimulation for several minutes helps to prevent and treat cardiovascular problems to relieve palpitations and angina. Relieves nausea and stops vomiting; treats anxiety, emotional pain and insomnia.*

P 7 DALING
In the middle of the crease on the underside of the wrist. *Treats anxiety and palpitations, carpal tunnel syndrome, wrist pain, and numbness of third and fourth fingers.*

P 8 LAOGONG
Where the nail touches the palm when the middle finger is flexed. *Calms a restless and disturbed mind; treats epilepsy, cardiac pain and hand pain.*

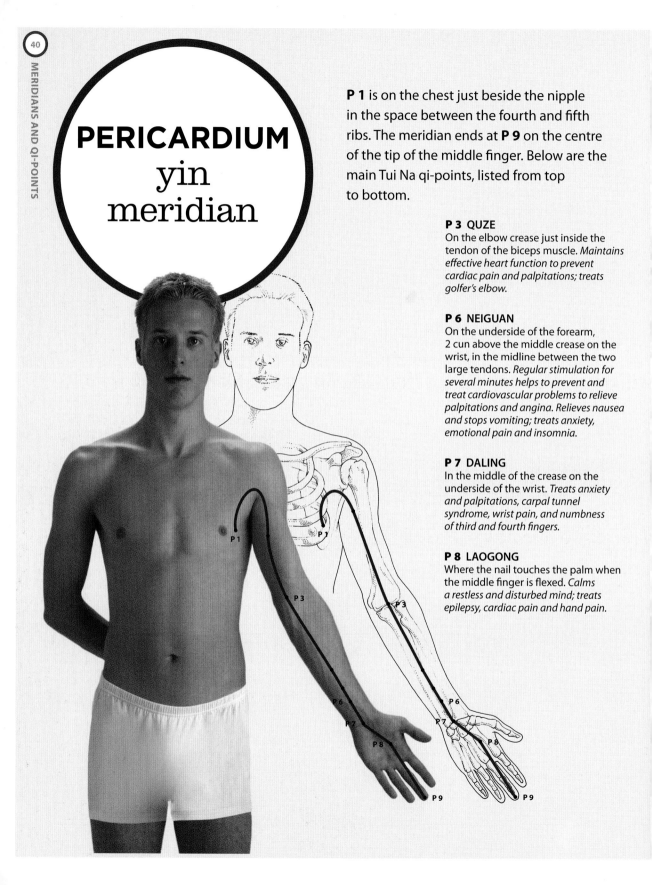

The meridian starts at **SJ 1**, on the outside of the fourth finger just behind the nail and ends at **SJ 23** on the outside tip of the eyebrow. Below are the main Tui Na qi-points, listed from top to bottom.

SANJIAO yang meridian

SJ 23 SIZHUKONG
In a depression at the outer tip of the eyebrow. *Improves eyesight; treats lateral headaches, muscle twitching in the eyelids and sore eyes.*

SJ 17 YIFENG
In a depression behind the ear lobe. *Treats tinnitus, deafness, facial paralysis and lower jaw neuralgia.*

SJ 15 TIANLIAO
1 cun below GB 21 or midway between SI 13 and GB 21. *Treats upper back and shoulder pain.*

SJ 14 JIANLIAO
In a depression just below the outer tip of the acromion on the back of shoulder joint. *Keeps the shoulder joint mobile; treats shoulder pain and immobility.*

SJ 10 TIANJING
In the depression approximately 1 cun above the base of the humerus when the elbow is flexed. *Treats elbow pain.*

SJ 5 WAIGUAN
2 cun up from the crease on the back of the wrist between the radius and the ulna. *Treats shoulder pain and immobility, forearm and wrist pain, lateral headaches, ear problems and flu.*

SJ 3 ZHONGZHU
In the depression between the fourth and fifth metacarpal bones just behind the knuckles. *Treats poor hearing and tinnitus, lateral migraine, and lateral neck and back of hand pain.*

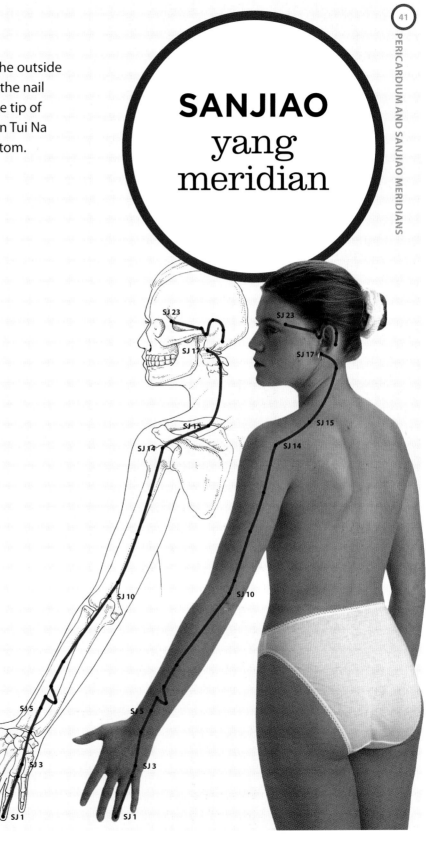

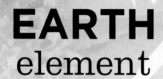

EARTH
element

The **spleen yin** and the **stomach yang** meridians are the **foot** yin/yang meridian partners and are each energetically linked to their named organ. Both are classified under the **earth element** in Five Element theory.

FUNCTIONS OF THE SPLEEN YIN ORGAN

CONTROLS PRODUCTION OF QI AND BLOOD FROM FOOD Weak spleen qi can result in extreme tiredness, abdominal bloating and loose stools.

DIRECTS QI AND FLUIDS UPWARDS TO THE LUNG Impaired spleen function results in oedema, heavy feeling in the limbs and mental lethargy due to excess dampness.

CONTROLS THE INTEGRITY OF THE BLOOD VESSELS Weak spleen qi function can cause heavy or prolonged menstrual bleeding, a tendency to bruise easily, varicose veins and oedema.

CONTROLS MUSCLES Weak spleen qi function causes weak, achy muscles.

HAS ITS CONNECTION WITH THE EXTERIOR THROUGH THE MOUTH AND LIPS Weak spleen qi can cause mouth ulcers and sore lips.

FUNCTION IS LINKED TO WORRY Spleen qi malfunction can cause obsessive thinking and affect the ability to concentrate, study and be creative.

SPLEEN YIN (SP) AND STOMACH YANG (ST) MERIDIANS

SPLEEN YIN MERIDIAN
Recommended qi-points for treatment:

- digestive problems SP 6, SP 4, SP 3, BL 20, LIV 13
- abdominal bloating SP 4, SP 3, SP 6, SP 15, BL 20, LIV 13
- oedema in the legs and ankles SP 9, SP 6, SP 3, BL 20
- big toe joint pain SP 3
- menstrual problems, infertility SP 6, SP 8, SP 10, BL 20, LIV 13
- poor sleep, worry SP 6, SP 4
- aching muscles throughout the body, fibromyalgia SP 21, LIV 13, BL 20

STOMACH YANG MERIDIAN
Recommended qi-points for treatment:

- headache ST 41, ST 8
- toothache ST 44, ST 7, ST 6
- jaw pain ST 7
- bloating, diarrhoea, constipation ST 36, ST 25, ST 21, BL 21, R 12
- pain in the knee ST 35
- front leg pain and hip pain ST 36, ST 31, ST 34
- difficulty conceiving ST 29, ST 25, ST 36
- boosting the immune system ST 36, BL 21, R 12
- obesity ST 36, ST 40, ST 25, ST 21

NOTE: problems on these foot meridians should be treated with Tui Na massage applied along them, with focused kneading of appropriate qi-points and related back shu points BL 20 and BL 21, and front mu points LIV 13 and R 12.

FUNCTIONS OF THE STOMACH YANG ORGAN

DIGESTS FOOD Any disturbance of stomach qi will adversely affect stomach function to cause stomach ache, nausea and maybe vomiting or hiccups.

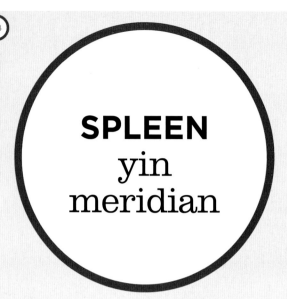

SPLEEN
yin
meridian

The spleen meridian starts at **SP 1**, on the outer margin of the big toe just behind the nail, and ends at **SP 21**, 6 cun below the armpit, between the sixth and seventh ribs. Opposite are the main Tui Na qi-points, listed from top to bottom.

SP 21 DABAO
Sits 6 cun below the armpit between the sixth and seventh ribs. *Boosts blood function to remove stagnation.*

SP 15 DAHENG
On the abdomen, level with, and 4 cun to the side of, the navel. *Improves bowel action.*

SP 10 XUEHAI
2 cun above the top edge of the kneecap on a vertical line drawn from the inner border of the kneecap. *Improves blood function; regulates bleeding in the menstrual cycle and spasming quadriceps muscle, and can relieve itchiness.*

SP 9 YINLINGQUAN
On the inside edge of the tibia, where the bone flares. *Treats local knee pain; reduces dampness in the tissues to prevent swelling; treats oedema and loose stools.*

SP 8 DIJI
5 cun below the medial knee eye. *Treats all menstrual problems.*

SP 6 SANYINJIAO
Just under the inside edge of the tibia, 3 cun above the tip of the inner ankle bone. *Stabilizes digestion; tonifies the three foot yin organs to improve sleep, boost energy, regulate menstruation, improve fertility and reduce dampness.*

SP 4 KUNGSUN
In the middle of the arch of the foot, just beneath the upper end of the first metatarsal. *Strengthens digestion, treats abdominal pain and insomnia, and regulates menstruation.*

SP 3 TAIBAI
In the arch of the foot, just beneath the lower end of the first metatarsal. *Strengthens spleen functions to improve digestion, tones muscle and clears the mind. Treats joint pain at the base of the big toe.*

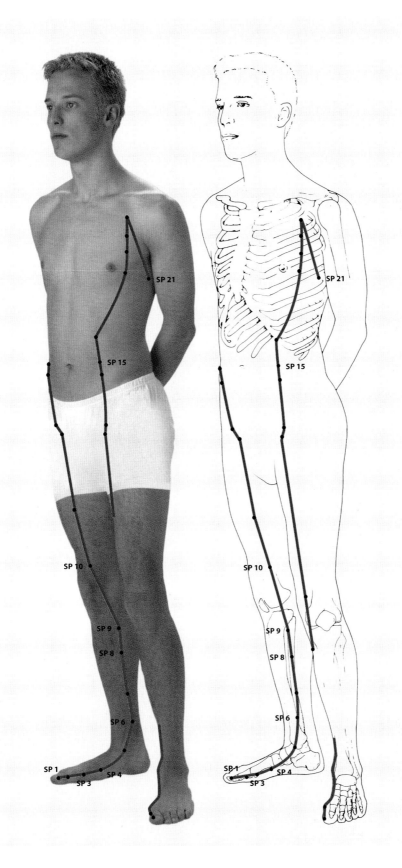

SP 21

SP 15

SP 10

SP 9

SP 8

SP 6

SP 1

SP 3   SP 4

SP 21

SP 15

SP 10

SP 9

SP 8

SP 6

SP 1

SP 3   SP 4

STOMACH
yang meridian

The stomach meridian starts at **ST 1**, just on the lower edge of the eye socket, in line with the pupil, and ends at **ST 45** on the outside of the second toe, just behind the nail. Opposite are the main Tui Na qi-points, listed from top to bottom. For **front mu** points, see page 26.

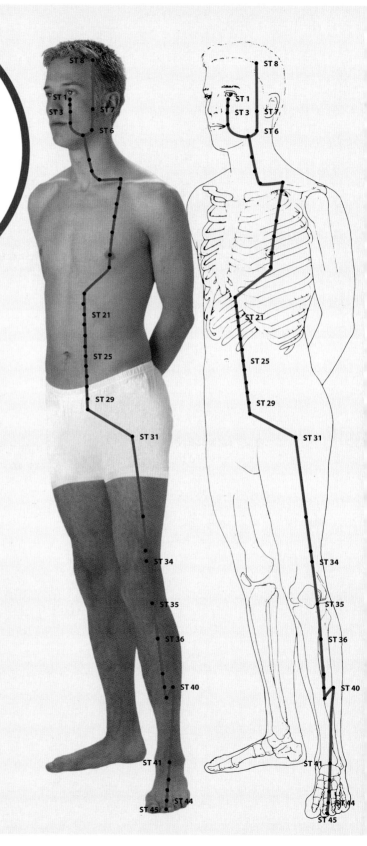

ST 3 JULIAO
Below ST 1, level with the nostril. *Maintains clear sinuses, benefits the eyes and treats facial paralysis.*

ST 6 JIACHE
In the middle of the jaw muscle, just above and in front of the angle of the lower jaw bone. *Treats toothache in the lower jaw and improves blood flow to the gums.*

ST 7 XIAGUAN
Directly above ST 6 in the notch between the jaw bone and cheekbone; easy to find if the mouth is opened and closed. *Improves blood flow to the gums of the lower jaw; treats jaw pain, upper jaw toothache, poor hearing and facial paralysis.*

ST 8 TOUWEI
4.5 cun from the midline of the forehead and 0.5 cun above the corner of the hairline. *Enhances blood flow to the head and treats eye disorders.*

ST 21 LIANGMEN
4 cun above the centre of the navel and 2 cun to the side of the midline. *Improves the stomach's digestive functions; treats abdominal muscle spasm, bloated abdomen and loose stools.*

ST 25 TIANSHU Large intestine mu
2 cun to the side of the centre of the navel. *Maintains healthy, normal bowel function; treats pain and bloating in the abdomen, diarrhoea, constipation and irregular menstruation.*

ST 29 GUILAI
4 cun below the centre of the navel and 2 cun to the side of the midline. *Improves fertility and regulates the menstrual cycle; treats prolapse of the uterus and hernia.*

ST 31 BIGUAN
On the thigh below the iliac crest, level with the lower border of the pubic bone. *Maintains tone in the rectus femoris; treats pain in the thigh.*

ST 34 LIANGQIU
2 cun above the intersection of two lines – one across the top edge of the kneecap and the other along its outer edge. *Relaxes the quadriceps muscles; treats knee and stomach pain.*

ST 35 DUBI
In a depression (lateral knee eye) below the outer edge of the kneecap. *Improves knee flexibility; treats knee pain.*

ST 36 ZUSANLI
3 cun below ST 35 and 1 cun lateral to the crest of the tibia. Strengthens the whole body's qi and immune system to boost vitality. *Improves digestion and treats stomach pain, diarrhoea and constipation, irregular menstruation and knee pain; strengthens the legs for easier walking.*

ST 40 FENGLONG
2 cun outside the crest of the tibia, halfway between the knee crease and the tip of the outer ankle bone. *Reduces the formation of phlegm in the tissues to aid weight loss; relieves mucus congestion in the lung.*

ST 41 JIEXI
In the middle of the front ankle crease. *Keeps ankle joints flexible; treats ankle joint pain, frontal headaches and abdominal bloating.*

ST 44 NEITING
Between the second and third toes just above the web. *Improves blood flow to the toes; treats toothache and aids weight loss.*

METAL
element

The **lung yin** and the **large intestine yang** are the **hand** yin/yang meridian partners and are each energetically linked to their named organ. Both are classified under the **metal element** in Five Element theory.

FUNCTIONS OF THE LUNG YIN ORGAN

CONTROLS THE PRODUCTION OF QI FROM AIR If lung qi is weak, you will feel tired, breathless and lacking vitality.

CONTROLS THE DISPERSAL OF BODY FLUIDS Weak lung function results in dry hair and skin and frequent, spontaneous sweating even when the body temperature is normal.

CONTROLS DEFENSIVE QI FUNCTIONS FOR THE SKIN, HAIR AND MUCOUS MEMBRANES If lung qi is weak, you can easily catch colds, flu and even develop asthma. The skin will become susceptible to infection and allergies such as dermatitis, impetigo and eczema.

PROMOTES BLOOD FUNCTIONS If this function is weak, it affects all the internal organs, as the circulation will be sluggish.

LUNG YIN (LU) AND LARGE INTESTINE YANG (LI)

LUNG YIN MERIDIAN
Recommended qi-points for treatment:

- coughs, colds, asthma **LU 9, LU 7, LU 6, LU 5, LU 2, BL 13, LU 1**
- sore throat **LU 7, LU 10, LU 11, BL 13, LU 1**
- front of the shoulder joint pain **LU1**
- thumb pain **LU 10**
- wrist pain **LU 7, LU 9**
- elbow pain **LU 5**

LARGE INTESTINE YANG MERIDIAN
Recommended qi-points for treatment:

- headache **LI 4**
- toothache **LI 4**
- runny or blocked nose **LI 20, LI 4**
- fever **LI 11**
- front of the shoulder joint pain **LI 15, LI 14, LI 4**
- tennis elbow **LI 11, LI 10**
- repetitive strain injury of hand or thumb **LI 4**
- pain in the body **LI 4**
- wrist pain **LI 5**

NOTE: problems on these hand meridians should be treated with Tui Na massage applied along them, with focused kneading of appropriate qi-points and related back shu points BL 13 and BL 25 and front mu points LU 1 and ST 25.

LINKS WITH THE EXTERIOR THROUGH THE NOSE Through this link, it's possible for external pathogens to gain access to the body if the lung qi is weak, resulting in a runny or blocked nose.

LINKED TO THE GRIEF EMOTION Weak lung function results in an inability to complete the grieving process.

FUNCTIONS OF THE LARGE INTESTINE YANG ORGAN

HELPS CONTROL WATER BALANCE The lung and large intestine interact to ensure good fluid distribution and balance. If too much water is absorbed, the result is constipation. If too little water is absorbed, the result is diarrhoea.

LUNG yin meridian

The lung meridian starts at **LU 1**, level with the space between the first and second ribs and 6 cun from the midline. It ends at **LU 11** on the outside of the thumb. Below are the main Tui Na qi-points, listed from top to bottom. For **front mu** points, see page 26.

LU 1 ZHONGFU Lung front mu
Below LU 2, level with the space between the first and second ribs. *Strengthens the lung to improve qi extraction from the air; treats coughs, chesty colds and asthma.*

LU 2 YUNMEN
In a depression just under the outer end of the collarbone, 6 cun from the chest midline. *Promotes respiration; treats coughs.*

LU 5 CHIZE
On the elbow crease just outside the tendon of the biceps muscle. *Strengthens lung function to resist infections and allergies, treats dry coughs, sore throat, fever and elbow pain.*

LU 7 LIEQUE
On the thumb side, 1.5 cun above the wrist crease, just above the bony lump (styloid process) on the radius. *Boosts immunity to prevent colds; relieves flu symptoms, coughs, headache and reduced neck mobility; helps withdrawal from smoking.*

LU 9 TAIYUAN
On the main wrist crease just inside the large tendon that runs down to the thumb. *Strengthens all lung functions and treats coughs and asthma; treats wrist weakness and pain.*

LU 10 YUJI
Just under the midpoint of the first metacarpal bone (at the base of the thumb). *Treats sore, dry throats, fever and thumb pain.*

LU 11 SHAOSHANG
At the outside margin of the thumb just behind the nail. *Treats sore, swollen throat.*

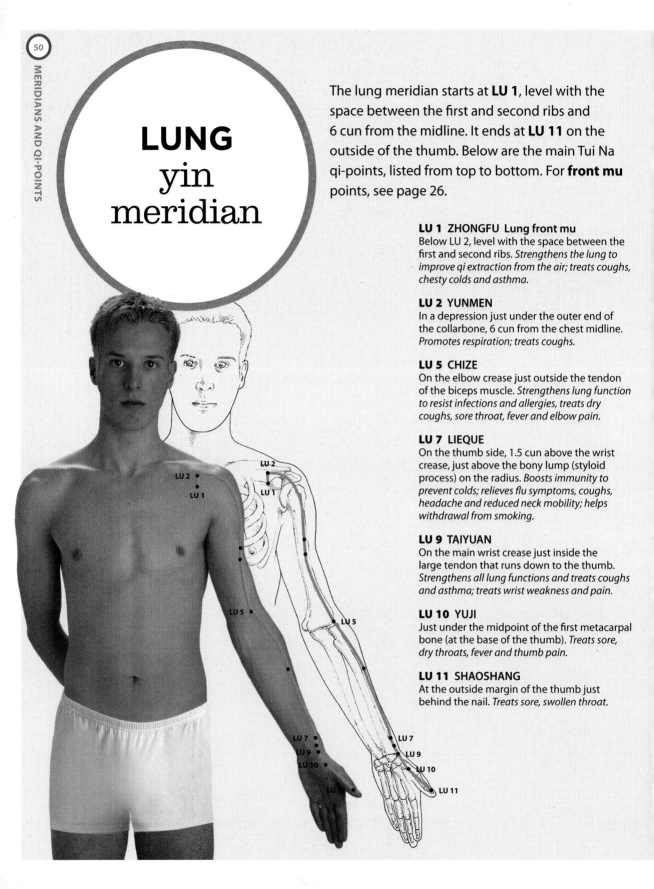

Starts at **LI 1** on the thumb side of the index finger just behind the nail, and runs along the arm to the face, ending at **LI 20** on the outside of the nostril on the opposite side. Below are the main Tui Na qi-points, listed from top to bottom.

LARGE INTESTINE
yang meridian

LI 20 YINGXIANG
In the depression on the side of the opposite nostril. *Maintains a clear nose and good sense of smell; treats nasal discharge and congestion, sinusitis and rhinitis.*

LI 15 JIANYU
In a depression just below the front, top edge of the shoulder bone (acromion). *Maintains shoulder mobility; treats shoulder pain and immobility.*

LI 14 BINAO
On a line from LI 11 to LI 15 level with the lower end of the deltoid muscle. *Maintains good tone in the deltoid muscle and treats upper arm pain in the deltoid region.*

LI 11 QUCHI
At the outer end of the elbow crease when the arm is flexed. *Regulates blood pressure; maintains elbow joint mobility and treats tennis elbow; reduces heat to treat fever, sore throats and itchy skin; balances digestion.*

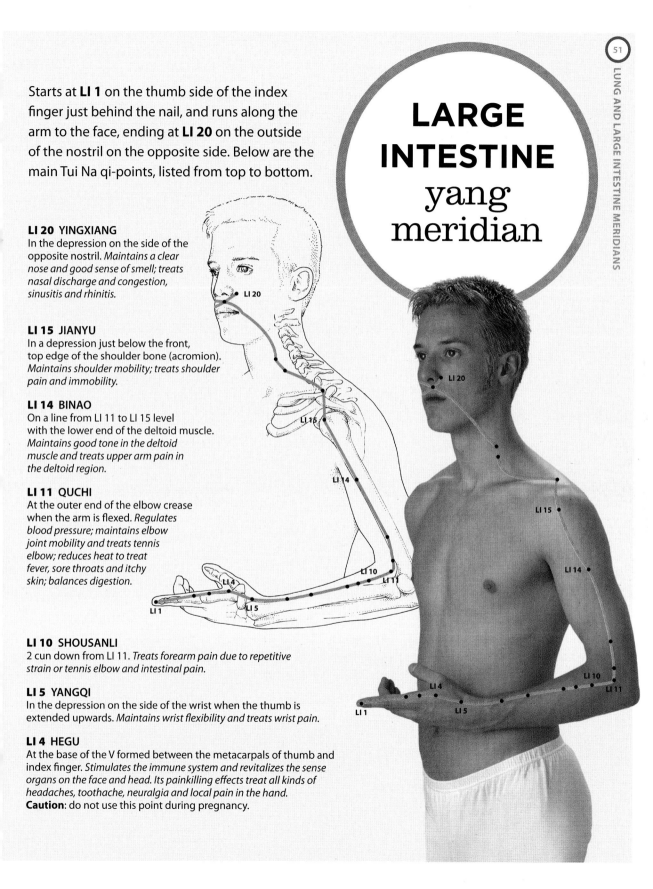

LI 10 SHOUSANLI
2 cun down from LI 11. *Treats forearm pain due to repetitive strain or tennis elbow and intestinal pain.*

LI 5 YANGQI
In the depression on the side of the wrist when the thumb is extended upwards. *Maintains wrist flexibility and treats wrist pain.*

LI 4 HEGU
At the base of the V formed between the metacarpals of thumb and index finger. *Stimulates the immune system and revitalizes the sense organs on the face and head. Its painkilling effects treat all kinds of headaches, toothache, neuralgia and local pain in the hand.*
Caution: do not use this point during pregnancy.

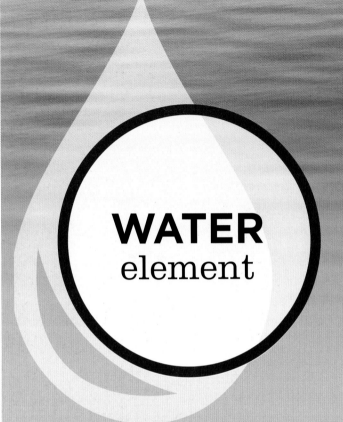

WATER
element

The **kidney yin** and the **bladder yang** are the **foot** yin/yang meridian partners and are each energetically linked to their named organ. Both are classified under the **water element** in Five Element theory.

FUNCTIONS OF THE KIDNEY YIN ORGAN

CONTROLS THE RESERVES OF JING AND QI FUNCTION Weak kidney jing function reduces resistance to disease, can cause impotence, infertility and lack of sexual desire, and increases the likelihood of old age marred by health problems.

CONTROLS THE PRODUCTION OF 'MARROW' FOR HEALTHY BONES AND BRAIN Chronic kidney weakness causes achy back and knees, osteoporosis, dental problems, memory loss and ultimately Alzheimer's and dementia.

REGULATES WATER BALANCE Failure of the kidney to remove excess water leads to oedema (swelling of the tissues, with excess fluid in the ankles and feet) and fluid congestion of the lung.

THE KIDNEY RECEIVES AND HOLDS QI FROM THE LUNG Weak kidney function prevents the efficient retention of qi from the lungs, causing asthma, breathing problems and reduced resistance to external pathogens.

HAS ITS CONNECTION WITH THE EXTERIOR THROUGH THE EARS Weak kidney qi can cause poor hearing and tinnitus.

CONTROLS THE LOWER ORIFICES Kidney qi weakness leads to bladder and anal incontinence, premature ejaculation, seminal emission and vaginal discharge.

MAINTAINS HEALTHY HAIR GROWTH Weak kidney jing results in early greying and thinning hair.

KIDNEY IS LINKED TO THE FEAR EMOTION Weak kidney function results in an inability to handle situations that involve fear.

FUNCTIONS OF THE BLADDER YANG ORGAN

STORES AND EXPELS WASTE FLUID Weak kidney qi or invasion by external pathogens, such as cold and damp, disturbs normal bladder function to cause frequent and profuse urination.

KIDNEY YIN AND BLADDER YANG MERIDIANS

KIDNEY YIN MERIDIAN
Recommended qi-points for treatment:

- lower back pain **K 1, K 3, K 13, GB 25**
- insomnia **K 1, K 3**
- tranquillizing the mind **K 1**
- poor hearing **K 3, K 6**
- coughs **K 25, K 27**
- oedema **K 7**
- back of the knee pain **K 10**
- medial ankle pain **K 3**
- cold hands and feet **K 1, K 3**
- urinary problems **K 3, K 7, K 10, BL 28, K 13**

BLADDER YANG MERIDIAN
Recommended qi-points for treatment:

- lower back pain **BL 22, BL 23, BL 24, BL 25, BL 26, BL 54, BL 37, BL 40, BL 57, BL 60, GB 25**
- sacroiliac pain **BL 26, BL 27, BL 28**
- hamstring pain **BL 36, BL 37**
- calf muscle pain **BL 57**
- back of the knee pain **BL 40**
- outer ankle pain **BL 60**
- neck pain **BL 10**
- eye problems **BL 1, BL 2**
- fertility issues **BL 32, BL 23**
- urinary problems **BL 23, BL 28, R 3**
- problems with internal organs – use the back shu points on the bladder meridian (**BL 13, BL 14, BL 15, BL 18, BL 19, BL 20, BL 21, BL 23, BL 25, BL 27, BL 28**) and front mu qi-points (see page 26)

NOTE: problems on these foot meridians should be treated with Tui Na massage applied along them, with focused kneading of appropriate qi-points and related back shu points BL23 and BL 28, and front mu points GB 25 and R 3.

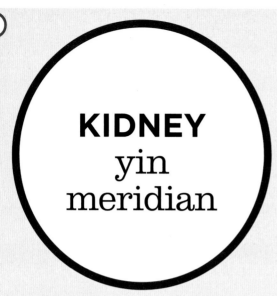

KIDNEY
yin
meridian

The kidney meridian starts at **K 1** on the sole of the foot and ends on **K 27** just under the collarbone, 2 cun from the midline. Opposite are the main Tui Na qi-points, listed from top to bottom.

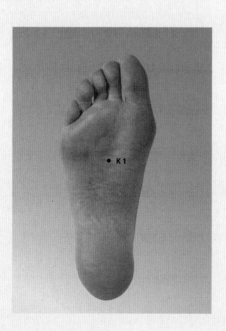

• K 1

K 27 SHUFU
Just under the collarbone, 2 cun from the midline. *Improves kidney/lung interaction for effective breathing; treats chronic coughs, coughs with phlegm and chest congestion.*

K 25 SHENCANG
Between the second and third ribs, 2 cun out from the midline. *Treats coughs, asthma and chest congestion.*

K 13 QIXUE
2 cun above the pubic bone and 0.5 cun lateral to the midline. *Treats lower back pain and supplements R 4 to strengthen the lower back.*

K 10 YINGU
On the inner end of the crease, behind the knee. *Maintains knee flexibility to prevent arthritis; treats medial knee swelling and pain, lower back pain and urination problems.*

K 7 FULIU
2 cun directly above K 3. *Maintains fluid balance between lymph and blood to prevent and treat oedema and daytime sweating.*

K 6 ZHAOHAI
In a small depression directly below the centre of the inner ankle bone. *Treats the same conditions as K 3, as well as a dry cough and night sweating.*

K 3 TAIXI
Midway between the tip of the inner ankle bone and the Achilles tendon. *Strengthens all kidney functions for strong lower back, good hearing and high fertility; treats frequency of urination and insomnia.*

K 1 YONGQUAN
On the midline of the sole, two-thirds along from the back of the heel. *Calms the mind for good sleep and lowers blood pressure; cools hot feet and treats painful soles, fainting and epilepsy.*

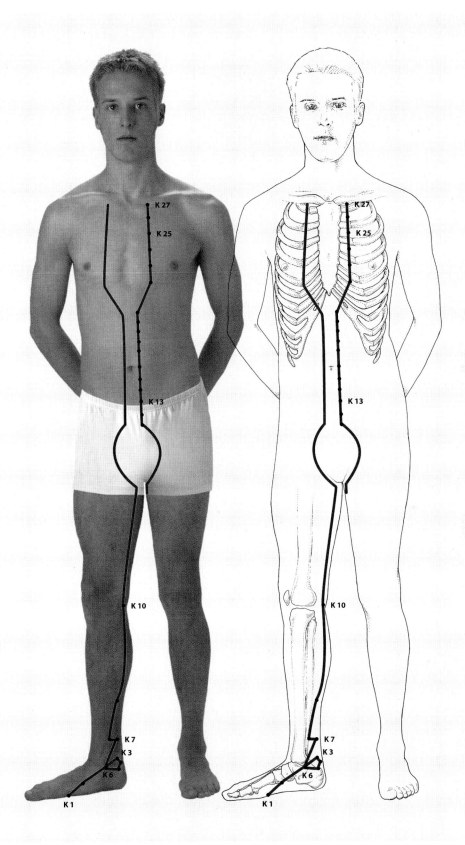

BLADDER
yang meridian

This is the longest meridian.
BL 1 is on the inner eye corner and
ends at **BL 67** on the outer edge of
the little toe, just behind the nail. Below
are the main Tui Na qi-points, listed from
top to bottom. The **back shu** points are
on this meridian (see page 26). The outer
bladder meridian runs 3 cun lateral to
the midline between **BL 41** and **BL 54**.

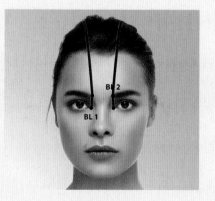

BL 2 ZANZHU
On the inner tip of the eyebrow. *Maintains
eye health; treats nasal congestion and
frontal headache.*

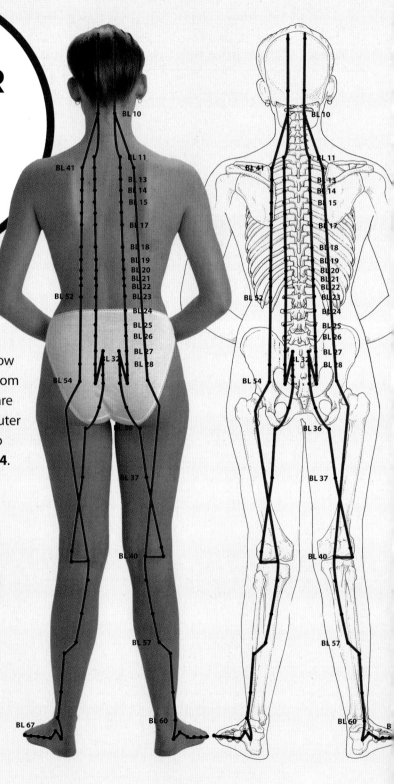

BL 10 TIANZHU
1.3 cun to the side of the midline, just below the base of the skull. *Deep kneading relaxes tense neck muscles, easing pain and headaches; treats inability to turn the head.*

BL 11 DASHU
1.5 cun from the midline, level with the lower border of the spinous process of thoracic vertebra one. **Influential point for bones.** *Helps clear qi blockages in the neck, shoulder and upper back.*

BL 13 FEISHU Lung back shu
1.5 cun from the midline, level with the lower border of the spinous process of thoracic vertebra three. *Promotes healthy lungs for resistance to airborne infections; treats coughs, colds, nasal congestion and asthma.*

BL 14 JUEYINSHU
Pericardium back shu
1.5 cun from the midline, level with the lower margin of thoracic vertebra four. *Complements the effects of BL 15 to improve the functions of the heart organ to slow the onset of cardiac disease.*

BL 15 XINSHU Heart back shu
1.5 cun from the midline, level with the lower border of the spinous process of thoracic vertebra five. Promotes heart function for a calm relaxed mind, good memory and a healthy, physical heart; treats insomnia, palpitations and heart conditions such as angina; treats shoulder pain and tension headaches.

BL 17 GESHU
1.5 cun from the midline, level with the lower border of the spinous process of thoracic vertebra seven. **Influential point for blood.** *Nourishes blood function; treats all kinds of blood problems involving bleeding and itchy skin conditions.*

BL 18 GANSHU Liver back shu
1.5 cun from the midline, level with the lower border of the spinous process of thoracic vertebra nine. *Regulates liver qi and blood to remove stagnation; maintains flexibility of joints, calms the emotions, relieves upper abdominal pain, benefits eye health and lowers blood pressure.*

BL 19 DANSHU
Gall bladder back shu
1.5 cun from the midline, level with the lower margin of thoracic vertebra ten. *Complements the effects of BL 18, and together they promote healthy tendons and ligaments to maintain healthy spinal mobility.*

BL 20 PISHU Spleen back shu
1.5 cun from the midline, level with the lower border of the spinous process of thoracic vertebra eleven. *Promotes the healthy digestion and assimilation of food to improve energy and muscle tone; relieves tiredness and indigestion; improves fluid balance to treat diarrhoea and oedema.*

BL 21 WEISHU Stomach back shu
1.5 cun from the midline, level with the lower border of thoracic vertebra twelve. *Complements the effects of BL 20.*

BL 22 SANJIAOSHU
Sanjiao back shu
1.5 cun from the midline, level with the lower margin of lumbar vertebra one. *Strengthens the lower back; maintains fluid balance to reduce dampness.*

BL 23 SHENSHU Kidney back shu
1.5 cun from the midline, level with the lower margin of lumbar vertebra two. *Nourishes the bones, spinal cord and brain; strengthens the lower back and knees; improves hearing and memory.*

BL 24 QIHAISHU Sea of qi
1.5 cun from the midline, level with the lower margin of lumbar vertebra three. *Strengthens qi for a healthy lower back.*

BL 25 DACHANGSHU
Large intestine back shu
1.5 cun from the midline, level with the lower margin of lumbar vertebra four. *Strengthens and treats the lower back; relieves sciatica; regulates the function of the colon; treats diarrhoea and constipation.*

BL 26 GANYUANSHU Gate of yuan qi
1.5 cun from the midline, level with the lower margin of lumbar vertebra five. *Strengthens and treats the lumbar and sacral regions to maintain a flexible spine; treats sciatica.*

BL 27 XIAOCHANGSHU
Small intestine point
1.5 cun from the midline, level with the first sacral foramen (hole). *Treats sacroiliac pain and sciatica; improves digestion.*

BL 28 PANGGUANGSHU
Bladder point
1.5 cun from the midline, level with the second sacral foramen. *Treats sacroiliac pain, sciatica and urination problems.*

BL 32 CILIAO
In the second of the four pairs of foramina (holes) on the sacrum. *Relaxes the sacral muscles, eases lumbago and promotes fertility.*

BL 36 CHENGFU
In the middle of the crease below the buttock. *Relaxes and treats the hamstrings; relieves sciatica.*

BL 37 YINMEN
On the midline of the back of the thigh, 6 cun below BL 36. *Strengthens and treats the lower back; treats sciatica and hamstring pain.*

BL 40 WEIZHONG
At the midpoint of the crease behind the knee joint. *Maintains healthy knees and lower back; treats knee and lumbar pain.*

BL 52 ZHI SHI
3 cun to the side of the midline and level with BL 23. *Reinforces functions of BL 23.*

BL 54 ZHIBIAN
3 cun to the side of the midline and level with the fourth pair of foramina (holes) on the sacrum. *Essential for the health and treatment of the lower back and sciatica.*

BL 57 CHENGSHAN
In the centre of the calf, halfway between BL 40 and the outer ankle bone. *Relaxes and treats the calf muscles; treats lower back pain and relieves haemorrhoids.*

BL 60 KUNLUN
In the depression between the outer ankle bone and the Achilles tendon. *Treats lateral ankle pain, and heel and Achilles problems; relieves occipital headaches and lower back pain.*

REN yin meridian

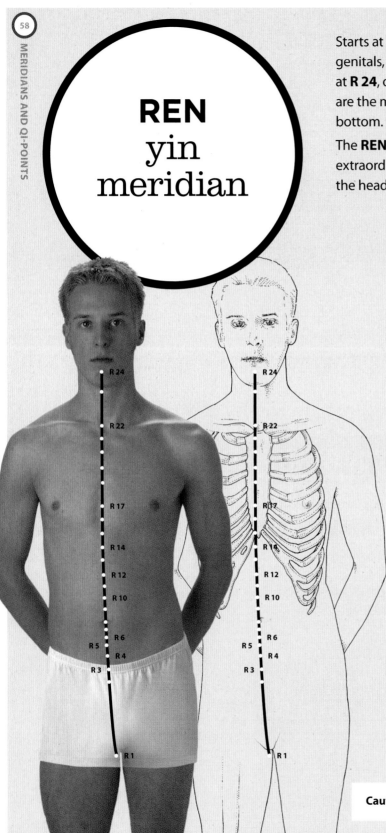

Starts at **R 1**, midway between the anus and the genitals, and runs up the front of the body to end at **R 24**, on the midline below the lower lip. Below are the main Tui Na qi-points, listed from top to bottom. For **front mu** points, see page 26.

The **REN** and **DU** meridians are the two single, extraordinary meridians that together encircle the head and trunk along the midline.

R 22 TIANTU
On the lower edge of the large depression at the top of the sternum. *Five minutes of strong finger kneading stops coughing and eases sore throats.*

R 17 TANZHONG Pericardium front mu
On the sternum, level with the space between the fourth and fifth ribs (in men, level with the nipples). *Reinforces the pericardium to maintain physical heart health; treats cardiac pain, asthma and coughing and has a calming effect.*

R 14 JUQUE Heart front mu
6 cun above the navel. *Regulates heart function to prevent blood stagnation and promotes good sleep; treats angina and palpitations.*

R 12 ZHONGWAN Stomach front mu
4 cun above the navel. *Promotes healthy digestion; treats gastric pain, vomiting and hiccups.*

R 10 XIAWAN
2 cun above the navel. *Strengthens stomach qi for good digestion.*

R 6 QIHAI
1.5 cun below the navel. *Translates as 'sea of qi'; intensifies all the body's qi functions.*

R 5 SHIMEN Sanjiao front mu
2 cun below the navel. *Regulates fluid balance for normal urination and colon function.*

R 4 GUANYUAN Small intestine front mu
2 cun above the pubic bone. *Promotes absorption and assimilation of food to tonify qi in the kidney, spleen and liver organs to improve overall energy, drive and fertility.*

R 3 ZHONGJI Bladder front mu
1 cun above the pubic bone. *Strengthens the urinary system; treats frequency and retention; boosts fertility, treats reproductive system problems and impotence.*

Caution: do not use **R 3** and **R 4** during pregnancy.

DU 1 is midway between the tip of the coccyx and the anus. The meridian ends at **DU 28**, inside the mouth at the junction of the gum and upper lip. Below are the main Tui Na qi-points, listed from top to bottom.

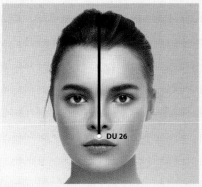

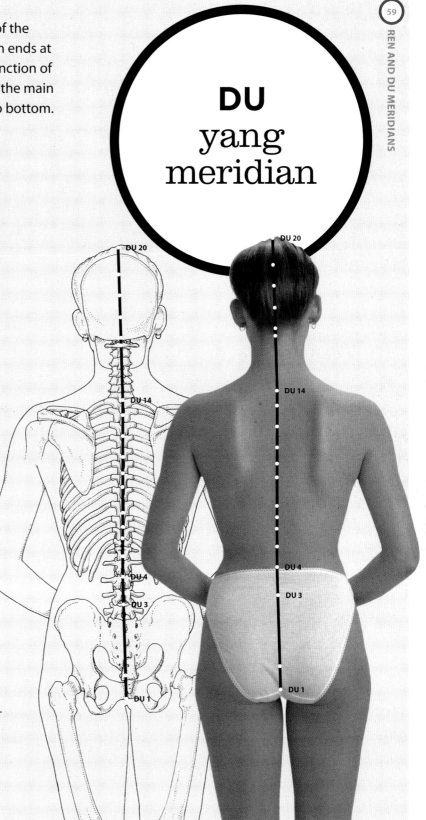

DU yang meridian

DU 26 RENZHONG
Two-thirds of the way up the furrow between the nose and lip. *Restores consciousness.*

DU 20 BAIHUI
At the top of the head, in a tiny depression, midway between the ears. *Calms the mind and promotes brain function; treats local headaches and dizziness.*

DU 14 DAZHUI
In the midline between cervical vertebra seven and thoracic vertebra one. *Balances the six yang meridians that meet here to strengthen qi and yang energies; treats fever and epilepsy.*

DU 4 MINGMEN
In the midline between lumbar vertebrae two and three. *'Mingmen' means 'gate of life' and strengthens the kidney to tonify the lower back.*

DU 3 YAOYANGGUAN
In the midline between lumbar vertebrae four and five. *Strengthens the base of the spine and legs.*

DU 1 CHANGQIANG
In the midline between coccyx tip and anus. *Treats haemorrhoids, difficult defecation and urination and anal pain.*

TUI NA TECHNIQUES

• • • • • • • • • • • • • • • • •

*This chapter describes the techniques used in
Tui Na and the particular effects of each one.
You will need to use these techniques in the
whole-body routine described in chapter 5.*

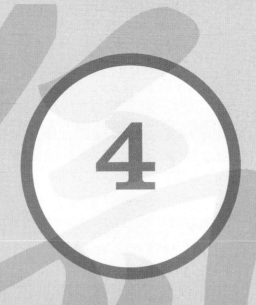

4

To familiarize yourself with the techniques, study the photographs and read the instructions in the following pages. You can then go on to practise the techniques either on yourself or on a partner, who should be seated comfortably in an upright chair or lying on a firm surface. Take turns to practise on each other, so that you know how it feels to receive Tui Na as well as to give it. Through practising these techniques with a partner, you will become sensitive to the finer nuances of Tui Na and to the feel of normal and dysfunctional tissues.

The 'soft tissue' techniques, which work on the muscles and underlying tissues, are presented first, on pages 63–71. Techniques for joint manipulation follow on pages 72–79. All these techniques stimulate the flow of qi and blood in different ways.

Before you start to practise Tui Na, consider whether your partner has any problems that contraindicate the treatment. If your partner has a condition that prevents you massaging directly on some of the qi-points, you can use distant points to achieve a good treatment.

WHEN NOT TO USE TUI NA

- Tui Na should not be applied directly to areas affected by skin cancer or the lymph node areas on those with lymphatic cancer.
- Do not use strong pressure or manipulations on anyone with brittle bones (osteoporosis), particularly the spine.
- Do not use Tui Na on the hip or knee area where an artificial joint is fitted.
- Avoid massaging directly on inflamed, bruised or broken skin, or over skin conditions such as eczema, psoriasis or shingles.
- During pregnancy, do not massage the lower back or abdomen or use qi-points SP 6 or LI 4.

Soft tissue techniques

All the techniques act on meridians and their qi-points, stimulating qi and blood flow to release blockages in the same way as acupuncture does. The aim of the soft tissue massage techniques is to apply pressure to the meridians and their qi-points to affect underlying tissues – muscles, ligaments, tendons and blood vessels. This pressure is applied in a variety of ways: at right angles to the body; in a circular motion; or with a shearing motion across the underlying muscles. The most important benefits of Tui Na are listed below.

BENEFITS OF TUI NA TECHNIQUES

- Moves and enhances qi and blood flow through the meridians.
- Releases qi and blood blockages to remove pain.
- Focused massage on qi-points changes the qi status of the meridian to provide specific health benefits.
- Promotes lymphatic drainage to prevent or reduce oedema.
- Releases fibrotic muscle fascia for muscle relaxation.
- Releases fibrotic subcutaneous connective tissue.
- Warms the underlying tissues to promote healing.

HOW TO APPLY PRESSURE

Begin every technique with fairly gentle pressure and increase it gradually, releasing it progressively as you finish. Interact with your partner throughout and be guided by any reaction. When you first start pressing a tense, knotted muscle, it may be uncomfortable. Only with repeated firm, concentrated pressing and kneading will the muscle release its tension and the pain subside as blood and qi-flow are re-established. Always be ready to reduce the pressure you use, or change to a different technique. In Tui Na, if the qi-points being massaged are tender, this can highlight a problem on that meridian and in the related organ.

Apply the pressure by leaning into your working arm with your body weight. The amount of pressure can be varied enormously, depending on the part of your body you use, and the amount of body weight you lean into the movement. To feel this, sit in an upright chair and press with your whole hand on your thigh. Then, without changing the amount of force, move your hand so you press just with the thumb. Using your thumb, you are pressing over a smaller area, so the pressure is greater. If you rock the thumb to and fro, keeping the end of it pressed on one point, or if you rotate the heel of the palm over a point, you apply a different kind of pressure again. Always alternate between right and left hands to develop equal strength, and do not rely on your dominant hand. For some of the steps in the sequence, the techniques are described for one side of the body only. To treat the other side, reverse right and left in the instructions.

The techniques are presented in groups. Within each group there are variations. For example, for kneading you can use the whole hand, the finger and thumb, or both hands interlocked. In the techniques that follow, 'you' refers to the giver, and 'your partner' means the receiver.

Kneading

This technique is fundamental to all Tui Na soft tissue techniques. Kneading must move the underlying tissues to create a range of different pressures, delivered with subtle nuances of direction and force. Kneading is achieved in a variety of ways by combining simple kneading with squeezing, rubbing and plucking techniques.

Using the thumb, heel of the hand, elbow or forearm, a skilled therapist can knead with the right amount of pressure on the area treated. Kneading may be to and fro or circular, or both. It can produce gentle, relaxing pressure or deep stimulation. When kneading, progress steadily from light to heavier pressure, guided by your partner's response.

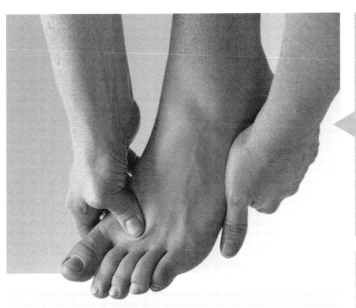

SINGLE THUMB KNEADING The thumb moves in a circle or to and fro to apply a penetrating pressure; the rest of the hand supports the thumb. Thumb kneading applies a very concentrated stimulus to a qi-point or a knotted area of soft tissue. For more focused pressure, use your nail tip (nailing) on the qi-points at the start and end of meridian lines on the fingers and toes (such as **LU 11** for an inflamed, sore throat).

DOUBLE THUMB KNEADING Press the other thumb down on top of the working one when stronger pressure is required.

HEEL OF THE THUMB KNEADING On the face, the Chinese use the fleshy area at the base of the thumb with a very loose side-to-side wrist action. The qi-point **LU 10** in the centre of this area is called 'fish belly'. It's softer than kneading using the thumb or heel of the hand.

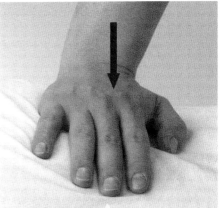

DOUBLE HEEL OF HAND KNEADING For even stronger pressure, place your other hand on top of the first to apply extra pressure. Bring your body weight over the hand to generate pressure, gently at first.

HEEL OF HAND KNEADING This uses the heel of one hand with the fingers relaxed on your partner's body. Pressure is focused through the heel, not the palm or fingers. Move the heel of the hand to and fro or in a circle. This technique covers a larger area than thumb kneading but with less focused pressure.

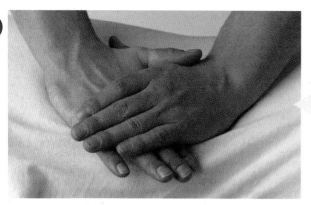

CROSSED DOUBLE HEEL OF PALM KNEADING With the heels of both hands pressing on the body, cross the fingers of one hand over the other. Lean into the body to give greater pressure with more precise control. Most frequently used on the bladder meridian on the back and legs.

SIDE-BY-SIDE HEEL OF PALM KNEADING With both heels of the palms side by side, use both hands simultaneously to apply pressure to massage the bladder meridian on the back or the thighs.

ELBOW KNEADING This technique uses the back of the elbow, not its tip, with to and fro or circular motion. It's used on well-muscled areas, such as the hips, buttocks, thighs, shoulders and lower back. Increase the pressure gently, since very deep pressure can be generated if too much body weight is used.

Elbow kneading is usually used on qi-point GB 30 on the buttocks, and BL 23–BL 26 on the lumbar area. It can also be used on GB 21, if your partner is big.

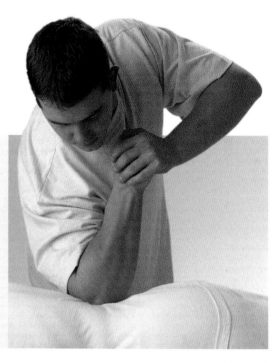

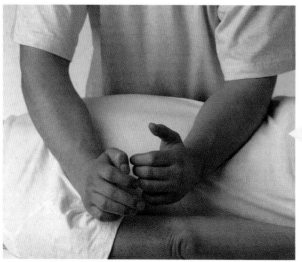

FOREARM KNEADING For less penetrating pressure, use the upper forearm. Here, both forearms knead simultaneously in opposite directions. Both elbow and forearm kneading are good for buttock and thigh massage.

Use this technique on the back, covering the whole spine, and working from the centre outwards and back again. Give a push on the outwards movement to effect a slight stretch.

Kneading with squeezing

The 'Tui' in 'Tui Na' means pushing or kneading. The 'Na' translates as a grasp that involves squeezing. In a squeeze, the tissues are held in a way that subjects them to pressures from opposite directions. Every squeeze lifts up and kneads the area being massaged. As for all techniques involving deep pressure, you should begin the squeeze gently and increase it gradually.

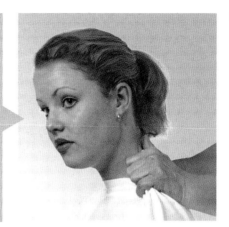

WHOLE HAND KNEAD WITH SQUEEZE Place the thumbs where you start the squeeze. The fingers press towards the thumb and heel of the palm, creating opposing pressures. Each squeeze involves a lifting action with kneading.

Use both hands simultaneously to give greater coverage.

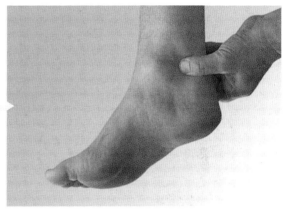

FINGER AND THUMB KNEAD WITH SQUEEZE A squeeze uses the thumb and all the fingers to give added strength to oppose the thumb pressure – for example, **BL 60** and **K 3**; **H 3** and **LI 11**; **SP 10** and **ST 34**.

This squeeze and knead produces deep and concentrated pressure on specific qi-points.

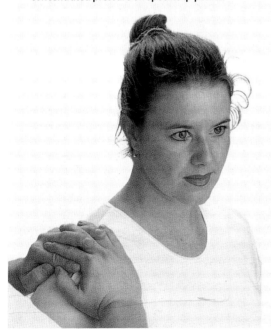

HEELS OF PALMS KNEADING AND SQUEEZING IN OPPOSITION Placing one hand on either side of the limb being treated, squeeze and knead with the heels of the hands, using strong opposing pressure with to and fro or circular movements. You can interlock your fingers if the location permits. This is good for the temples, shoulders, knees and ankles.

Kneading with pushing

Pushing is kneading firmly, but with the movement in one direction only, sufficient to move the underlying tissues. Pushing techniques are deep and vigorous.

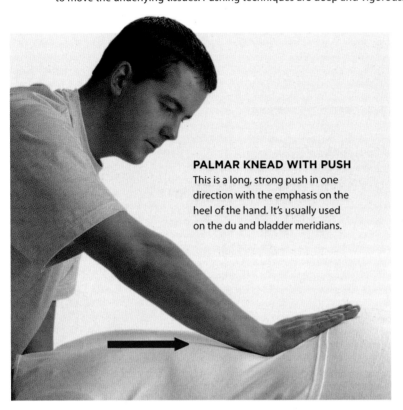

PALMAR KNEAD WITH PUSH
This is a long, strong push in one direction with the emphasis on the heel of the hand. It's usually used on the du and bladder meridians.

THUMB KNEADING WITH A PUSH Both thumbs push outwards from the midline. This is used on the face.

Kneading with thumb rocking

This technique applies penetrating thumb pressure on qi-points, to produce acupuncture-like effects.

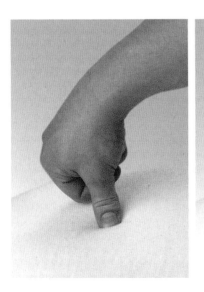

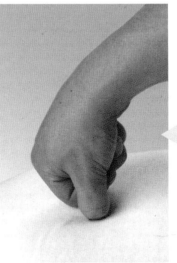

First make sure your thumb nail is short. Put your thumb pad on the area or qi-point to be treated and, with a small to and fro movement of the forearm, rock your hand over the thumb so that it bends at the first joint. The overall effect is to bend and straighten the thumb rapidly while holding it on the same spot to knead the underlying tissue. This technique should be done for several minutes on each qi-point.

Kneading with plucking

This technique uses a shearing action, with very deep, controlled, sideways movement across specific qi-points and muscles to move the underlying tissues. It's effective on the inner bladder meridian and GB 21.

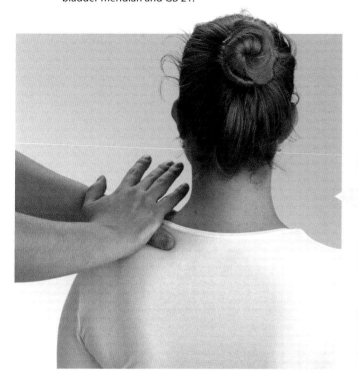

Place the thumb pad flat on the area being treated. Now use the heel of the other hand to push the thumb backwards and forwards, creating a kneading effect. Plucking works very well on qi-points over muscles that are tightly knotted.

Vibration

For this technique, the hand quivers, gently moving the underlying tissue and sending vibrations into them.

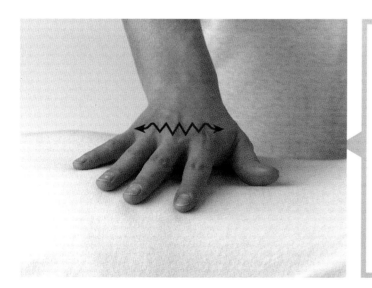

Holding your palm flat on your partner's body, tense the muscles in your forearm while keeping your fingers loose, so that your hand quivers. This technique is used mainly on the abdomen.

Rolling

Rolling is a modern technique, only introduced last century, but it's effective and important in Tui Na. Since the technique is difficult to learn from a book, an alternative version to Chinese rolling is also described here, which you may find easier. This is the single or double forwards knuckle roll, developed by the author. In all versions of the technique, the rolling action moves the underlying tissues like kneading does.

CHINESE ROLLING In Chinese rolling, the back of the hand rolls over the body. Press the outside edge of the back of the hand firmly against your partner's body, fingers held slightly apart and relaxed, as shown below. Keeping your wrist relaxed, rotate your forearm so that your hand flips smoothly backwards. As your hand rolls across your partner's body, it opens, so that the metacarpal region behind the knuckles and each of the fifth, fourth and third knuckles in turn make contact with the body.

Lean into your hand with your body weight to create the pressure required. The roll must be smooth, with the hand always in contact with your partner's body. Do not allow the hand to flick up at the end of the roll. The return movement is also smooth, with the fingers loose, as if cradling an egg. Aim to make one complete movement per second. An expert moves the hand like a rolling pin, making about 130 rolls per minute.

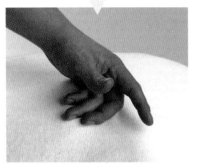

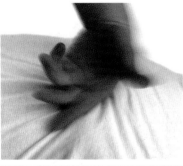

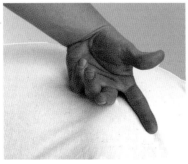

MARIA'S SINGLE KNUCKLE ROLLING Curl the fingers loosely, with the thumb relaxed, and put your hand on your partner's body, holding the top joints of the fingers and the nails against the area to be treated (see below). Roll the hand forwards, as far as the knuckles. Then retract the forearm so the hand rolls back into the original position.

This roll is a simple to and fro motion created by a piston-like action of the forearm. Each roll kneads the underlying tissues. Maintain an even pressure on the forward stroke as the backs of the fingers open out against the body. The hand should not rub or lose contact with the skin. This single roll is used down the inner bladder meridian from **BL11** to **BL 26**.

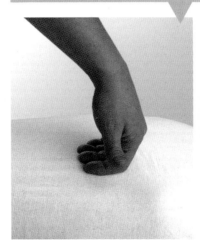

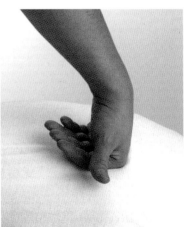

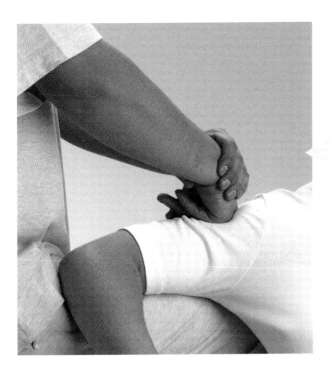

MARIA'S DOUBLE FORWARD KNUCKLE ROLLING With this roll, it's easier to control pressure than with the Chinese version. Place your free hand on top of the working one, which is more clenched than in the single roll. Only roll over your second finger joints as far as the knuckles. It's like a to and fro kneading action using the finger joints to strongly move the underlying tissues. The technique is used on the upper arm and across the bladder meridian towards the spine.

Rubbing

The Chinese describe rubbing techniques as pushing, scrubbing, chafing and dragging. Rubbing involves movement over the skin's surface, creating friction, which generates heat. The movements knead the subdermal tissues and can vary from a very gentle to and fro to a vigorous scrubbing.

ONE-HAND CHAFING This is rubbing with the outer edge of the hand, making long strokes with a fast sawing motion. The technique is used along the inner bladder meridian.

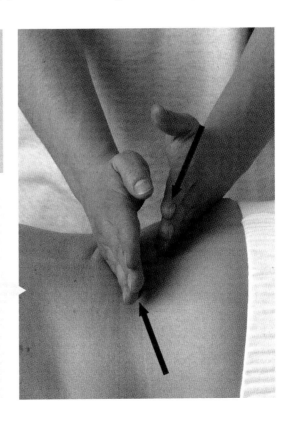

TWO-HAND CHAFING Here, both hands act like saws, moving in opposite directions with short, rapid strokes.

Chafing across the lumbar region warms and stimulates the kidney energies.

Chafing across the sacral area of the lower back generates heat that your partner may feel along the lines of the bladder meridian of the legs even as far as the feet.

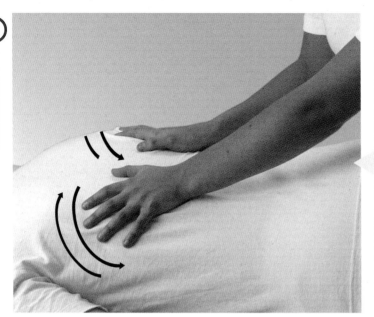

PALMAR RUBBING With a loose wrist action, use the whole palm to make light circular, or to and fro, fast rubbing movements to stimulate the subdermal tissues. Here, on the back, the hands move to cover the whole back. For stronger pressure, use the heel of the hand.

PALMAR RUBBING IN OPPOSITION This technique gives a vigorous rubbing with the palms on both sides of arms, legs, fingers, thumbs and shoulders.

Begin at the top of a limb and move downwards gradually.

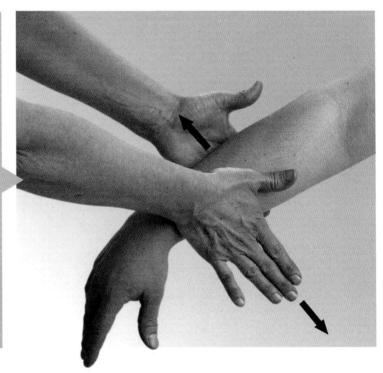

Percussion

Percussive techniques apply pressure for a very short time; the amount of pressure depends on the force used and the area over which it's applied. Percussion is mostly used to apply penetrating pressure to areas of the body with thick layers of muscle, such as the buttocks, the lumbar region, thighs and the muscles across the shoulders. Each technique produces a specific, therapeutic sound.

PUMMELLING Using the outer edges of loose fists, vigorously pummel your partner's body with a rapid staccato action. Alternate your hands as you pummel.

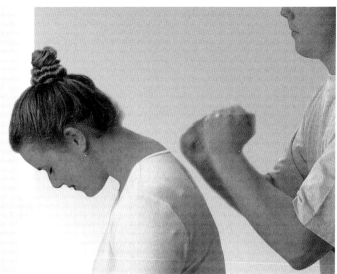

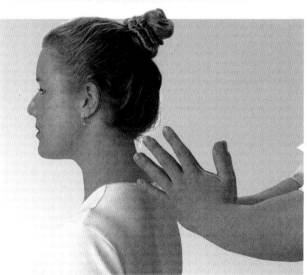

HACKING Hold the hands with palms together and fingers spread. Strike the body with the sides of the hands, with the emphasis on the little fingers so that the other fingers clap together.

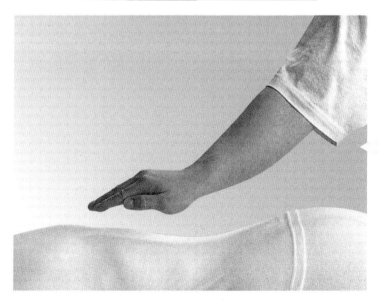

CUPPING Hold the hand firmly in a cupped position. Allow the forearm to drop loosely with each stroke, with the movement coming from the elbow. You can strike with some force because there is a cushion of air trapped between your hand and your partner's body. When cupping on the back, hold your hand across the sacral and lumbar area but lengthways along the spine itself. Use on well-muscled areas, such as **GB 30** and the thighs. The technique should produce a cushioned sound not a slap.

Joint manipulation techniques

Joint mobility can be maintained using joint manipulation techniques. These are safe for the treatment of stiff and aching joints, but always consider the physical limitations of the joint you are treating. The elbows and knees are mainly hinge joints, allowing movement in one plane, athough it's possible to get a little lateral movement in them. Only five joints in the body can rotate: two shoulders, two hips and the neck. Of these, only the shoulder joint can rotate in a full circle. The wrist and ankle are sliding joints. Always remember that manipulation involves leverage, which requires sensitivity. An effective stretch will just exceed what your partner would be normally capable of. Damage can easily result if the joint is overstretched.

To assess a joint problem, first ask your partner to move the joint as far as possible and tell you where there is stiffness or pain. Manipulate slowly and smoothly, and stop if you feel resistance.

Before using any joint manipulation techniques, use soft tissue massage on the qi-points around the joint. This stimulates qi and blood flow and relaxes muscles, tendons and ligaments, enabling you to work on the joint effectively.

These techniques relieve pain and obstruction in the joint capsule and the surrounding muscles. Contracted, tight muscles hold tension, which can be released by manipulation, allowing the muscles to lengthen and improve tone.

BENEFITS

- Stretches and manipulates the connective tissues of the joint capsule to aid joint mobility.
- Stretches the muscles that control the joint to improve muscle tone.
- Improves the distribution of qi and blood through the meridians into the joints.
- Removes qi and blood blockages from the meridians.

Shaking

The shake is used to treat the arms and legs. First loosen the muscles with a full soft tissue massage of the limbs. Shake only one arm at a time; the legs can be shaken individually or together.

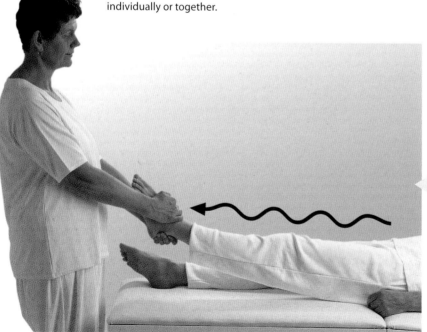

SINGLE LEG AND HIP SHAKE Lift the foot with one hand under the heel, grasping the top of the foot with your other hand, and pull gently.

Shake firmly ten times with small, rapid, up and down movements. Repeat five times.

The shake transmits through the hip and the spine for hip mobility. It eases pressure on the spinal nerves to relieve sciatica and hip pain.

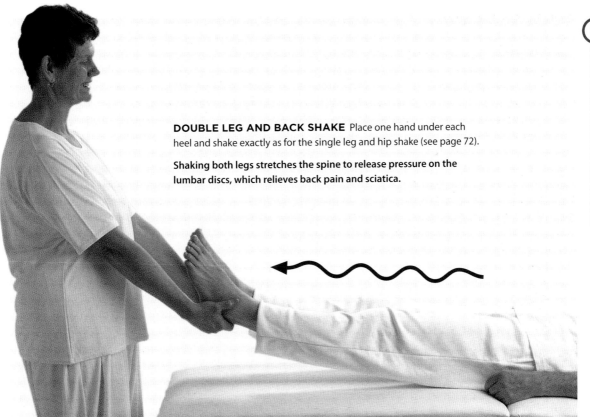

DOUBLE LEG AND BACK SHAKE Place one hand under each heel and shake exactly as for the single leg and hip shake (see page 72).

Shaking both legs stretches the spine to release pressure on the lumbar discs, which relieves back pain and sciatica.

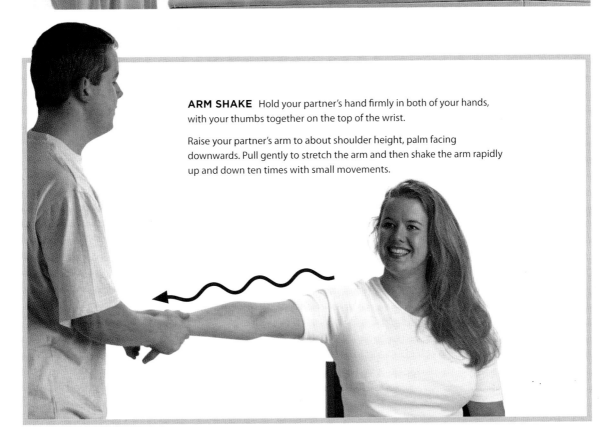

ARM SHAKE Hold your partner's hand firmly in both of your hands, with your thumbs together on the top of the wrist.

Raise your partner's arm to about shoulder height, palm facing downwards. Pull gently to stretch the arm and then shake the arm rapidly up and down ten times with small movements.

Extension and flexion

These techniques are used on hinge joints – the elbow and the knee.

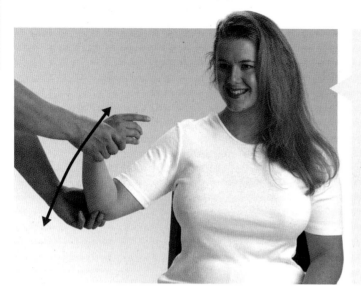

ELBOW EXTENSION AND FLEXION Flex your partner's arm, resting the elbow on your left hand, and press your thumb into **LI 11** (see page 51) and your middle finger into **H 3** (see page 38).

Holding your partner's wrist with your other hand, firmly flex and extend the arm, keeping your thumb and finger pressure on **LI 11** and **H 3**.

To increase the stimulation of the joint, rotate the forearm in both directions.

SUPINE KNEE EXTENSION AND FLEXION
Stand facing your partner's leg. Cupping one hand under the heel and resting the other over the kneecap, lift the leg into the position shown on the right.

Push the leg towards the body until you feel slight resistance. Now firmly extend the leg by pressing down on the knee while pulling the heel in the direction shown by the arrow. This manipulation improves flexibility in the knee and hip.

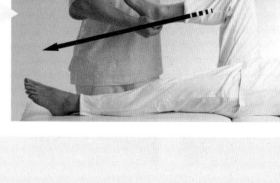

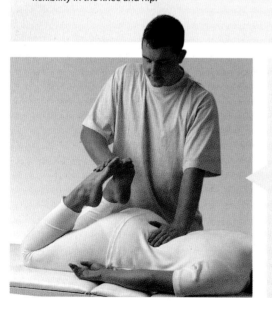

PRONE KNEE FLEXION Place your left hand over **BL 25** and **BL 26** and slide your other hand under the toes of both feet. Apply pressure on the lower back as you raise the feet to the buttocks.

Where there is extreme stiffness of the knee joint, flex one leg at a time. The lumbar press manipulates the back as well as the knees and hips for improved flexibility.

For a different effect, repeat with the lower legs crossed, each way in turn.

Rotation

In everyday life we don't use the full rotatory potential of our joints. Tui Na rotations help to compensate for this by improving joint mobility. Rotation techniques are used on the shoulders, hip joints, ankles and wrists. Neck rotations can cause serious injury and are not described in this book.

Always massage the soft tissues in the chosen area before attempting a rotation, to aid the flow of blood and qi and release muscle tension. With regular Tui Na, frozen shoulders and even joints affected by severe osteoarthritis can have their mobility improved.

SHOULDER ROTATION WITH ELBOW FLEXED
Stand behind your partner, supporting the right forearm on yours with a light grip under the wrist. With your other hand, grip the shoulder joint, pressing into **LI 15** (see page 51) and **SJ 14** (see page 41). Rotate the arm forwards and backwards. This gentle rotation releases shoulder pain and restriction. Each circular movement should be as large as the mobility of the joint will allow.

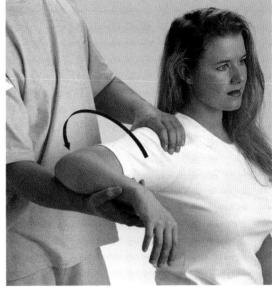

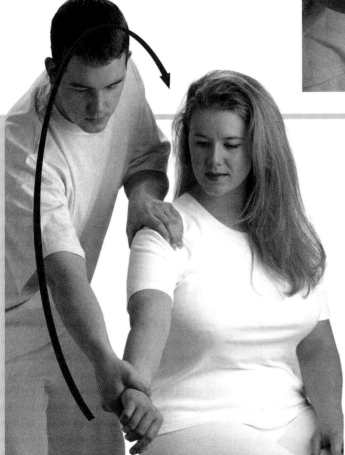

SHOULDER ROTATION WITH ELBOW EXTENDED Extend the arm, holding it loosely by the wrist. With your left hand, grip the shoulder joint, pressing **LI 15** (see page 51) and **SJ 14** (see page 41). Then rotate the arm slowly, with large circular movements, forwards ten times and then backwards ten times. Limit the size of the rotation if you feel any resistance.

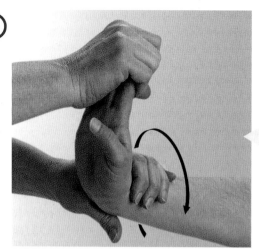

WRIST ROTATION With one hand, grasp the forearm firmly for support immediately above the wrist. With your other hand holding the fingers, rotate the wrist joint clockwise and anticlockwise, as far as possible. If someone has wrist pain, advise them to vigorously shake both wrists daily.

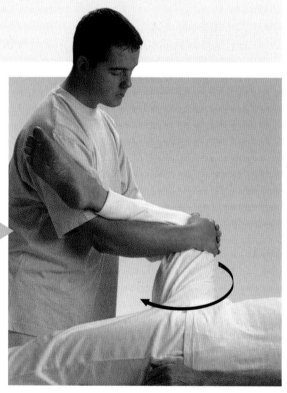

HIP ROTATION Flex your partner's right knee so that the lower leg is horizontal and supported across your right forearm, gripping the knee with interlocked hands. Use your hands to rotate the hip carefully, making clockwise and anticlockwise circles. Start gently and gradually increase the size of the rotations as far as the joint allows. Frequent, gentle rotations will improve mobility in arthritic joints.

Another method is to support the heel with one hand and use the other hand on the knee to guide the rotation. This is better for more flexible people, who need larger rotations.

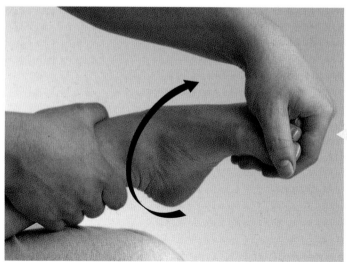

ANKLE ROTATION With your partner lying on their back, raise the foot a little, supporting it with one hand under the lower leg just above the ankle. With your other hand, grip the toes and rotate the foot clockwise and anticlockwise.

Pressing and stretching

These manipulations create two equal forces working in opposite directions: one force 'stretching' at a point distant from one force 'pressing'. The techniques flex and twist the joints to a greater degree than normal, improving their mobility. Carefully control the amount of force you use, feeling for any resistance. When you lift the shoulder or leg, the lumbar presses create a strong manipulation to align the spinal vertebrae.

SHOULDER STRETCH WITH LUMBAR PRESS With your partner lying face down, press your right hand firmly down on the lumbar region, with your heel over **BL 25/BL 26** on the left and your fingers resting on the spine.

Lean over and grasp your partner's right shoulder with your left hand. Now lift the shoulder while applying an equal but opposite force to the back. The result is a well-controlled but potentially vigorous stretch of the front shoulder and upper chest.

This technique gives a twist to the lumbar and lower thoracic spine to align the vertebrae. Repeat, readjusting your hand onto BL 23/BL 24.

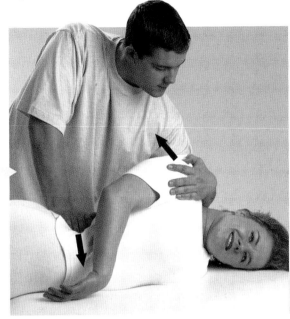

LEG LIFT WITH LUMBAR PRESS Standing on your partner's left, press your left hand onto **BL 26** on the side of the spine nearer to you. Slide your right hand under the left leg, holding it just above the knee, and lift the leg as far as is comfortable.

At the same time, press with equal force on the lumbar area. Hold the lift for a few seconds, rotating the leg slightly before lowering it.

Change sides and repeat on the other leg. Lifting the leg with sacrolumbar pressure aligns the sacroiliac joint.

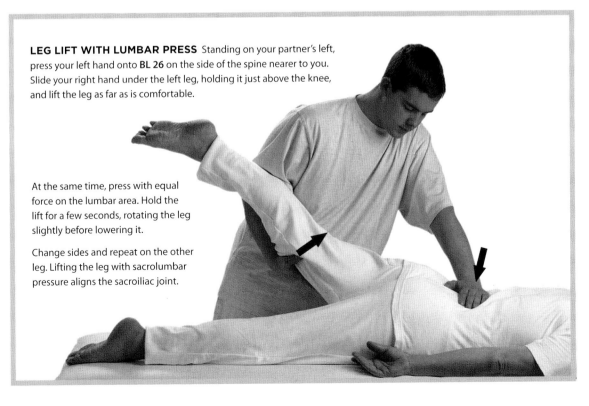

SHOULDER ROTATION STRETCH

Standing on your partner's left, lift the right arm, resting the forearm across the middle of the back. Lean over and slide your right hand under the elbow and up to the shoulder, and grasp it firmly. Your partner's elbow should lie on top of your forearm. Grasping the top of the shoulder with your left hand, rotate it slowly several times, starting with small movements and gradually making larger rotations, and give it a stretch.

This technique greatly facilitates qi-flow through the shoulders and into the arms, improving shoulder mobility.

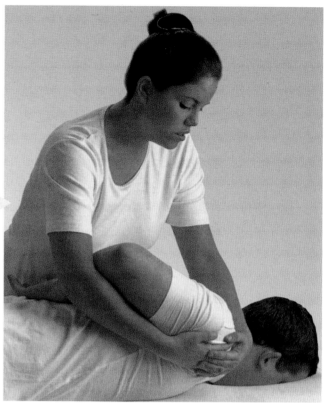

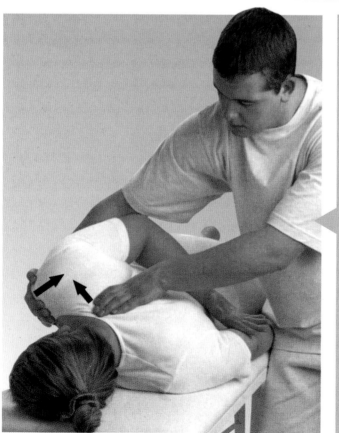

SHOULDER STRETCH WITH SCAPULAR PRESS
Raise your partner's shoulder with your right hand, keeping your left hand with your index finger and thumb pressed firmly against the inner edge of the right scapula, and simultaneously lift and press the shoulder against your left hand to give a powerful shoulder stretch.

Lift and press with equal force. Repeat, repositioning your hand along the scapula.

This technique stretches the front of the shoulder and presses the rhomboid muscles between the spine and scapula, easing tension in the upper back.

Stretching

This is a spinal stretch that eases back strain and relieves the pressure on damaged intervertebral discs. Even those who have no back problems find this stretch soothing and relaxing. Spinal stretches are excellent for opening the articular joints of the spinal vertebrae and relieving pressure on intervertebral discs. This improves spinal and sacroiliac flexibility.

STANDING SPINAL STRETCH Stand back to back with your partner, feet slightly apart, and link arms. With their buttocks above yours (flex your legs if necessary), bend forwards at the waist and lift your partner off the floor so the legs hang loosely. Shake your partner gently from side to side and lower slowly to the floor.

Caution: do not attempt this technique if you have back trouble, or with a partner much heavier or taller than yourself.

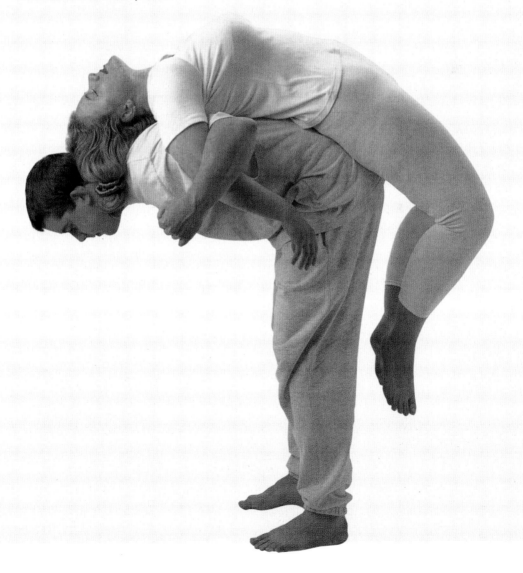

WHOLE-BODY ROUTINE

• • • • • • • • • • • • • • • • •

*The unique whole-body Tui Na routine described
in this chapter is a holistic treatment designed to
increase energy and vitality, and promote health and
well-being. This sequence of soft tissue techniques
and joint manipulations improves qi-flow, clearing
blockages and stagnation. The Chinese script on the
opposite page means qi. Unlike most other forms of
holistic massage, Tui Na has a sound basis in Chinese
medical theory. Clinically, it's used to treat many
different ailments and conditions.*

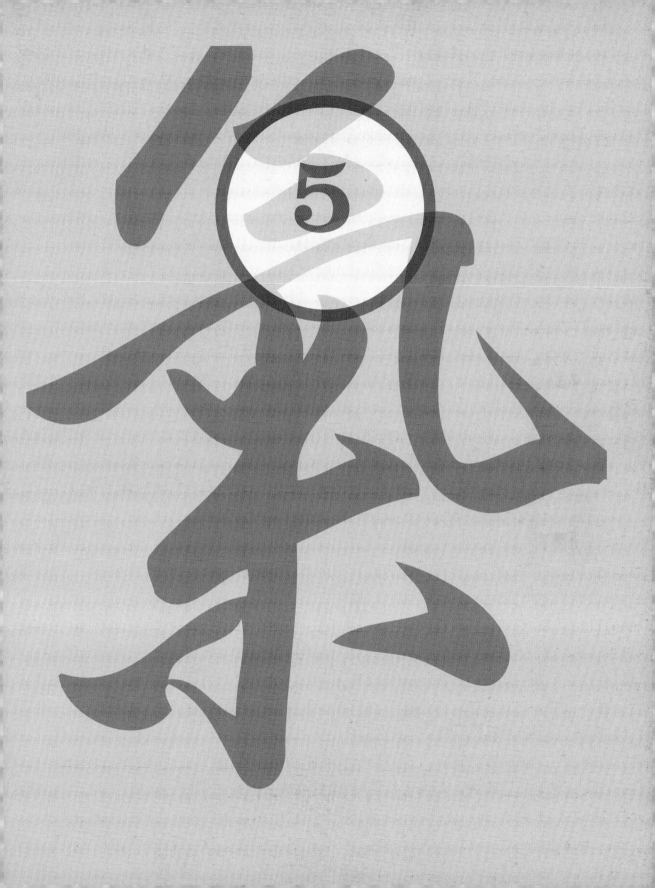

The routine presented here is a preventative treatment, which corrects any imbalances in the body's energy before symptoms and health problems can develop. Since, in traditional Chinese medicine, the body, mind and spirit are indivisible, the routine works very well to restore physical health, as well as emotional harmony.

When you first start to practise Tui Na, concentrate on the steps of the routine that use the simpler techniques: pressing, squeezing and kneading. Refer back to the descriptions of the techniques in chapter 4. For each step of the routine, an illustration shows you the meridians and qi-points used. This will also help you to visualize the meridians in the area you are massaging. For a fuller description of the positions and effects of the qi-points, refer to the relevant meridian illustration in chapter 3.

The whole-body routine is divided into seven parts, each concentrating on a different area of the body and with your partner in a different position. Work on each body area in the order shown, at least to begin with. When you are more experienced in giving Tui Na, you can concentrate on parts of the body that need specific treatments, as suggested in chapter 6. For example, you might give on-the-spot help to a partner suffering cramped muscles on the squash court, or a tension headache in the office, or even at a party. The routine described in this chapter, however, is meant to be carried out at home.

PREPARATION
To receive the full benefit from a Tui Na treatment the environment should be warm. For the first part of the routine, seat your partner in an upright chair with good back support. Later in the routine your partner will need to lie down on a comfortable flat surface, such as a massage couch. Have a few small cushions ready to support your partner during treatment. A bed is not suitable, as it's too low and will cause you back strain. If you don't have a massage table, you will need to do it on a floor padded with blankets.

You need to be able to move freely when giving Tui Na, so wear comfortable clothes and flat shoes, or go barefoot. Remove any rings and make sure that your fingernails are short. Your partner should wear soft clothes. A cotton T-shirt and tracksuit trousers are ideal.

Before you start the routine, prepare your partner by explaining what you are going to do and how it might feel. Tui Na is a vigorous and deep massage. Qi-points must be kneaded thoroughly, starting gently and increasing the pressure as you proceed. Encourage your partner to tell you if a qi-point is particularly painful. If so, it can indicate a problem somewhere on that meridian or in the related organ, and so additional kneading will be required to remove the stagnation. Observe all the cautions given in chapter 4.

Allow at least one hour for the routine. After a Tui Na treatment, your partner should feel relaxed but, at the same time, energized. Allow your partner time to unwind after the treatment, especially if there has been a release of emotional tension.

Throughout the routine the instructions are given for a right-handed person. If you are left-handed, you should reverse the positions given.

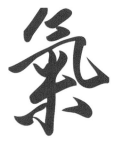

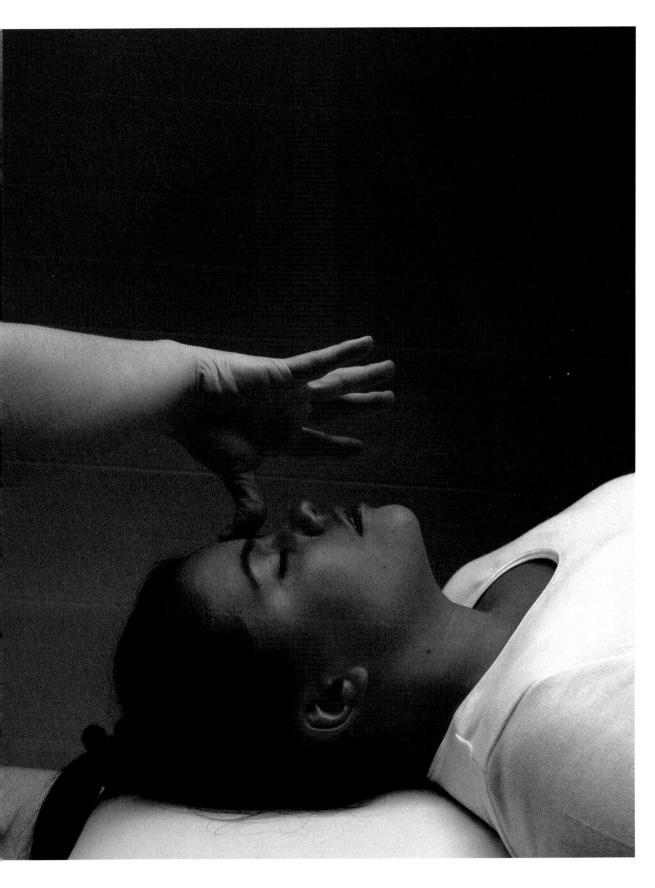

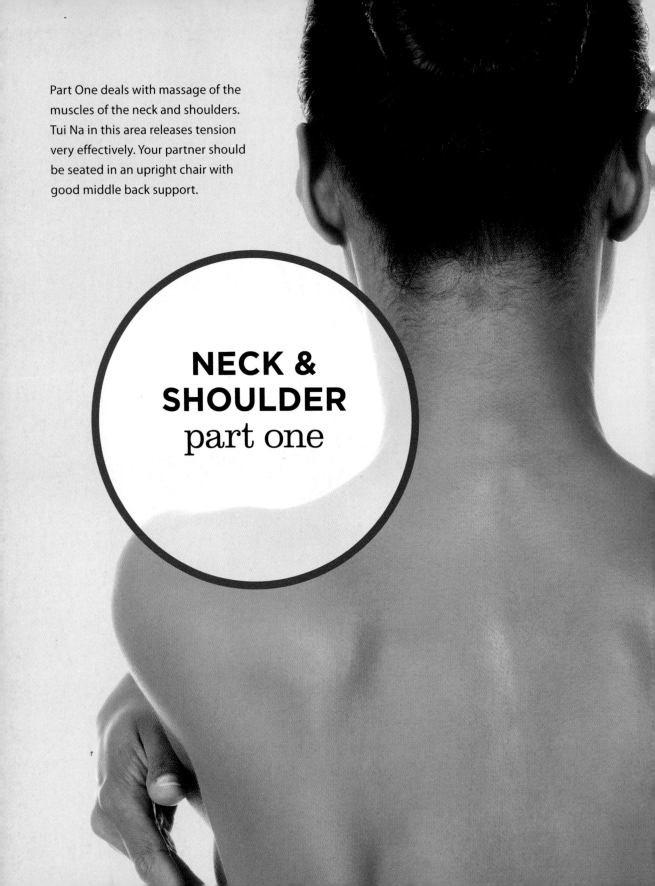

Part One deals with massage of the muscles of the neck and shoulders. Tui Na in this area releases tension very effectively. Your partner should be seated in an upright chair with good middle back support.

NECK & SHOULDER
part one

Main qi-points

The diagram below shows the qi-points that can be massaged when Tui Na is
applied to the neck and shoulders. These points are found on the following
meridians: bladder (blue), small intestine (red) and gall bladder (green).

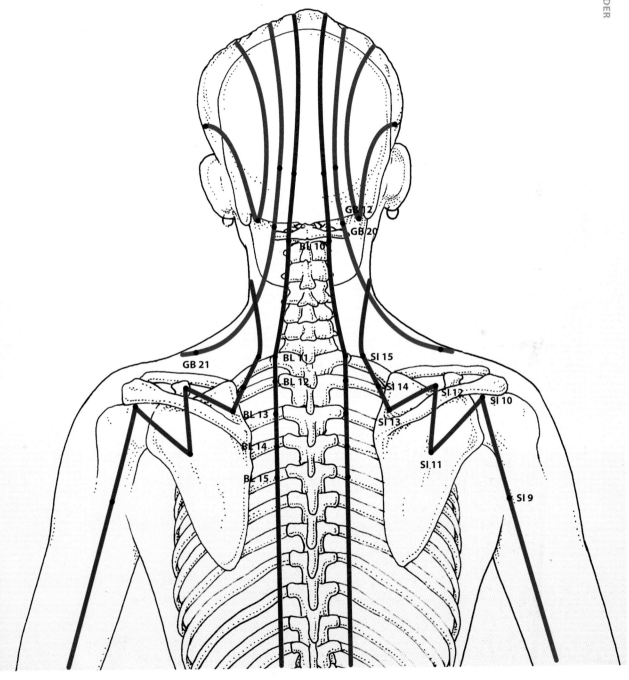

1 SQUEEZING AND KNEADING

Standing behind your partner, squeeze gently along the tops of the shoulders with the whole hand and then start heel of hand kneading. As the shoulders relax, feel for any tender qi-points or knotted tissues and thumb knead them thoroughly. Extend thumb kneading down both sides of the upper spine on the bladder meridian. Grasp the top of the shoulders and squeeze the muscles deeply.

These techniques unblock the energy channels from the head to the shoulders, releasing some of the layers of tension that so often accumulate across the shoulders.

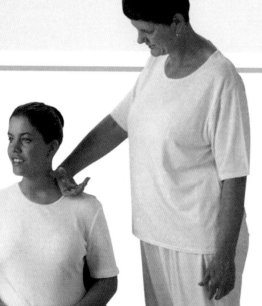

2 CHINESE ROLLING

Standing behind your partner's left shoulder, roll with your right hand along the muscles on top of the shoulder towards the base of the neck. Roll across this area for up to five minutes, concentrating on the gall bladder and small intestine meridians. Repeat on the right shoulder, using your left hand. Repeat this rolling often during the routine.

Rolling encourages the smooth flow of qi in the meridians, harmonizing the body's internal energy and creating a radiant feeling of well-being.

3 PRESSING AND KNEADING QI-POINTS

Repeat the squeezing and kneading of step 1, but now press and knead with the thumb on **GB 21, SI 9–15** and **BL 11–15**. Knead each point at least a hundred times.

Pressure applied to these qi-points may cause some discomfort, but this is necessary to release tension.

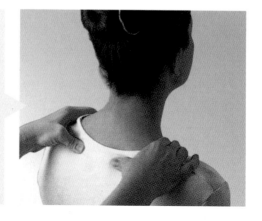

4 KNEADING BY PLUCKING ON THE SHOULDER

Place your left thumb on your partner's left **GB 21** with the fingers relaxed. Using the heel of your right hand over the left thumb, knead by plucking at least a hundred times across **GB 21**, pushing towards the neck. Repeat on the right shoulder.

Kneading by plucking GB 21 balances the energy flow to the head, relaxing shoulder and neck muscles and easing headaches. This simple method of relaxing knotted tissue gives a blissfully light feeling.

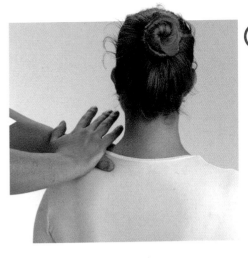

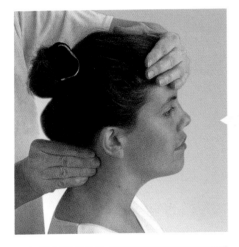

5 SQUEEZING AND KNEADING

Using your thumb and first two fingers, squeeze and knead the muscles on either side of the neck vertebrae with a definite kneading action, while the other hand lightly supports the forehead. Work from the base of the neck up to the region just beneath the skull, lifting the hand between each position. Change hands frequently.

This technique stimulates the bladder and gall bladder meridians, sweeping away the tension that leads to headaches and relieving stiff and aching neck muscles.

6 KNEADING QI-POINTS WITH PRESSURE

With the thumb and middle finger on **GB 20**, knead firmly with the pressure aimed upwards. Squeeze and knead each point at least a hundred times, then change hands and repeat. Now use the same technique on **BL 10**.

GB 20 is one of the best qi-points for treating all headaches and reducing blood pressure. It also affects the eyes, ears, nose and mouth. BL 10 relaxes stiff necks and can help tired and sore eyes.

7 PERCUSSION ON THE SHOULDERS

Use the pummelling technique on the top of the shoulders and either side of the spine between the shoulder blades. Hacking has a similar effect.

Pummelling is intensely exhilarating, as it moves both qi energy and blood.

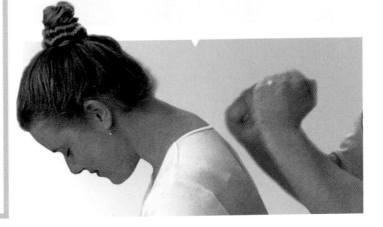

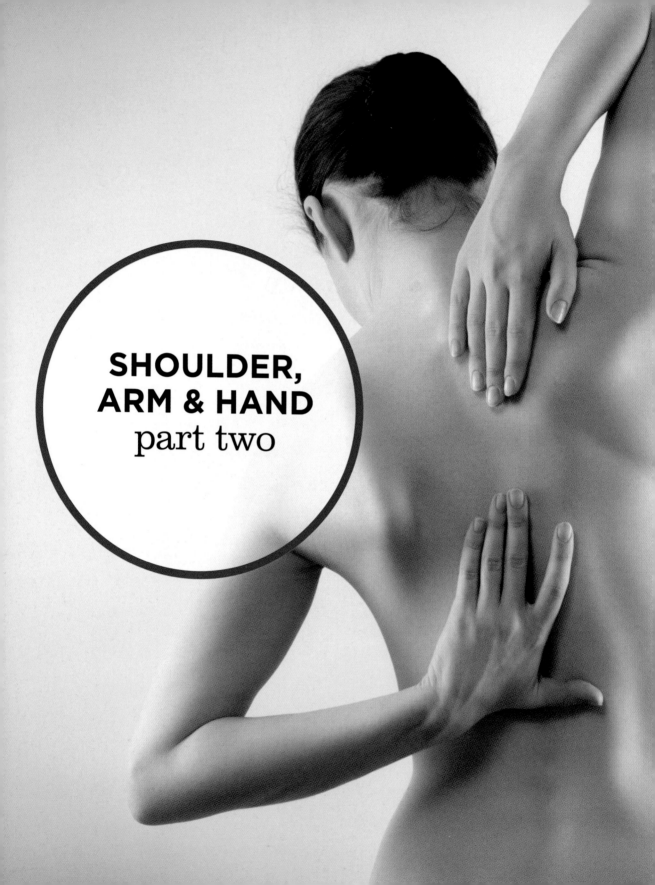

SHOULDER, ARM & HAND
part two

Main qi-points

The diagram below shows the qi-points that can be massaged when Tui Na is applied to the shoulder, arm and hand. These are found on the following meridians: sanjiao and small intestine (shown in red, on the left), large intestine and lung (grey), and the heart and pericardium (red, on the right). See more on meridians and individual benefits in chapter 3.

JIANQIAN – extra point

Midway between LI 15 and the armpit crease. Treats front arm pain.

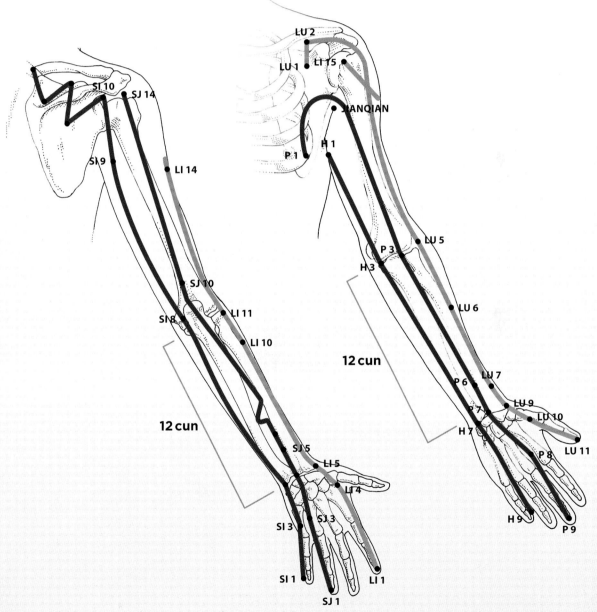

The first steps work on the right side of the body.

Position 1 Stand in front of the shoulder.
Position 2 Face the side of the shoulder.
Position 3 Stand behind the arm and face the back of the shoulder.

Repeat these three positions on the left arm.

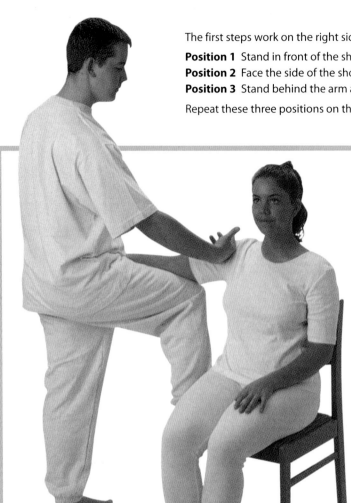

1 ROLLING THE FRONT RIGHT SHOULDER AND ARM

STAND IN POSITION 1 Standing on your partner's right, put your right foot on the chair so your thigh is about level with the armpit. With your left hand, grasp the right wrist and raise the arm so that it lies out across your knee. Turn your partner's wrist outwards from you to expose the deltoid muscle on the front shoulder. Roll with your right hand from **LI 11** and **LU 5** up this muscled area over **LI 15** to **LU 1** and **LU 2**. You can also roll up the forearm.

Rolling along the large intestine and lung meridians relieves tension and pain in the shoulders and arms.

2 SQUEEZING AND KNEADING THE FRONT OF THE RIGHT ARM

Grasping the muscle on the top of the shoulder with your right hand, squeeze firmly, pushing over the muscle and as you knead deeply between your fingers and the heel of your hand. Continue like this down the arm. Repeat this several times. Now squeeze and knead the tissues with the fingers and thumb lightly all the way down the arm, giving a slight lift between each position. Change hands frequently.

Squeezing and kneading relaxes shoulder and arm muscles.

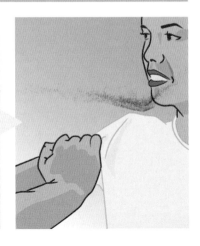

3 PRESSING QI-POINTS

With either hand, press into qi-points **LI 15** and **SJ 14** with your thumb and middle finger. Press and knead deeply with a rocking motion at least a hundred times, and for several minutes if there is any shoulder pain. Knead the extra point – **jianqian** – which is midway between **LI 15** and the front armpit crease. Thumb knead up and down the large intestine meridian, between **LI 15** and **LI 14**. Then knead **LU 1** and **LU 2**.

LI 15 and SJ 14 relax the muscles around the joint capsule to improve shoulder mobility. They relieve pain caused by injury or arthritis. Stimulating the lung meridian boosts qi in the lungs to relieve chest problems and cold symptoms.

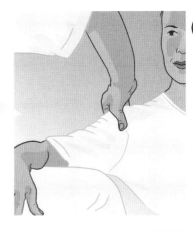

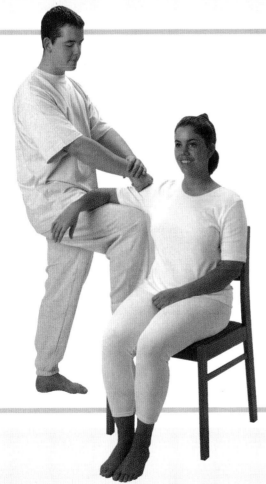

4 ROLLING THE TOP OF THE SHOULDER JOINT

STAND IN POSITION 2 Facing your partner's side, stand with your foot up and your knee facing the armpit. The upper arm is supported across your knee with the forearm bent. Use the double rolling technique on the deltoid muscle to the border of the shoulder bone. Roll for several minutes.

Rolling here boosts qi-flow in the meridians. LI 15 and SJ 14 ease pain when stimulated strongly.

5 SQUEEZING AND KNEADING THE TOP OF THE SHOULDER JOINT

Repeat the squeezing and kneading of step 2 on the upper arm but this time using each hand alternately. Your right hand squeezes and pushes the muscles of the arm backwards, and your left hand squeezes and pushes forwards.

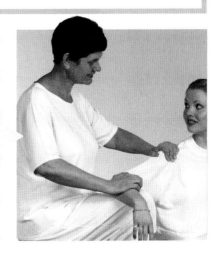

6 PRESSING QI-POINTS Repeat step 3.

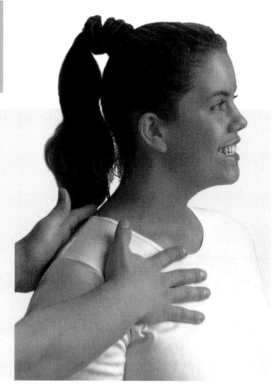

7 PALM RUBBING THE CHEST AND SHOULDER BLADES IN OPPOSITION

Place your right hand on the right upper area of your partner's chest and your left hand on the right shoulder blade, with your wrists and fingers relaxed. Palmar rub this area with brisk, alternate, light, up and down movements for at least one minute.

Stimulates the whole chest and targets LU 1 and LU 2. The technique relieves front shoulder pain and is good for asthma sufferers and those with coughs and other chest problems.

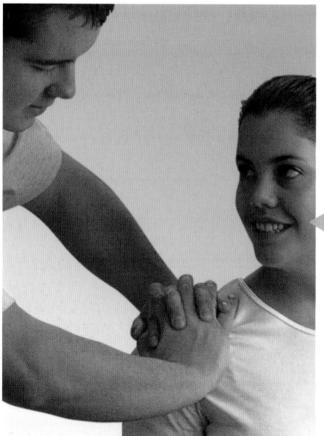

8 HEELS OF PALMS SQUEEZING AND KNEADING IN OPPOSITION

Place your hands across the top of your partner's right shoulder, with fingers interlocked and the heels of your hands tucked tightly into the hollows on the back and front of the shoulder (you may need to loosen your fingers to do this). Then knead deeply with the heels of both hands into **LI 15** and **SJ 14**, making circular movements, for about one minute.

Improves shoulder mobility and should always be used on any painful or 'frozen' shoulder.

9 RUBBING DOWN THE ARM

Support your partner's arm between your hands, just below the armpit. The arm should be completely relaxed. Palmar rub rapidly with alternating to and fro movements, massaging down the arm to the wrist (see right). Repeat several times.

Powerfully stimulates the flow of qi, in all the meridians of the arm to ease pain and tension.

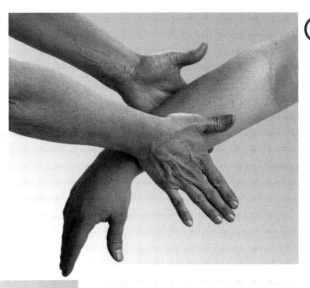

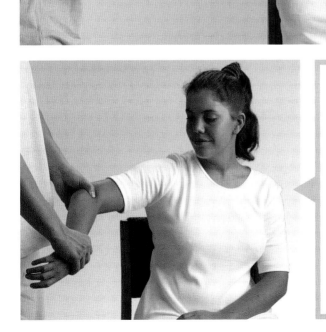

10 SHAKING THE ARM

Hold your partner's hand firmly with both your hands, with your thumbs together on the top of the wrist. Raise the arm to just below the horizontal and pull gently to loosen the shoulder joint. Then shake ten times with firm, rapid, small up and down movements. Repeat the shake five times.

Opens the joint capsule to improve shoulder mobility and relieve pain.

11 PRESSING AND KNEADING ARM QI-POINTS

Press and knead **LI 11** and **H 3** with the thumb and middle finger. At the same time rotate the forearm in both directions with your other hand, holding the wrist lightly. Press and knead **LI 11** and **LU 5**, **P 3** and **H 3** and **SJ 10**. Then press and knead **SJ 5** and **P 6** together, using your thumb and middle finger like pincers.

LI 11 with H 3 and LU 5 with P 3 treat elbow pain. P 6 with SJ 5 has a calming effect on the mind and emotions.

12 PRESSING AND KNEADING HAND AND WRIST

Hold your partner's wrist with both your thumbs on top and use your middle fingers under the palm and wrist to flick the hand upwards several times. Then press and knead points **LI 5, LU 7, LU 9, LU 10, P 7, P 6** and **H 7**.

Steps 12 and 13 stretch connective tissues in the wrist to improve flexibility, and to ease wrist pain and carpal tunnel syndrome.

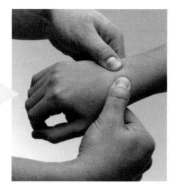

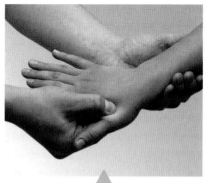

13 PRESSING AND KNEADING THE JOINTS

Using your index finger and thumb, firmly press and knead all the finger joints and knuckles in turn. Then press and knead **LI 4, LI 5, SJ 3, SJ 5** and **SI 3**.

Caution: do not use **LI 4** during pregnancy.

Hand and wrist massage presses some of the most powerful qi-points, increasing the overall feeling of well-being.

14 ROLLING THE BACK OF THE SHOULDER JOINT

STAND IN POSITION 3 Stand behind your partner, with your right foot on the chair, holding the wrist with your right hand so the right arm is across your knee. Turn the hand and arm forwards to expose the back of the shoulder joint. Now roll over this area with your left hand. Roll over **SJ 14, SI 9, SI 10** and **SJ 10** and then roll down the exposed forearm.

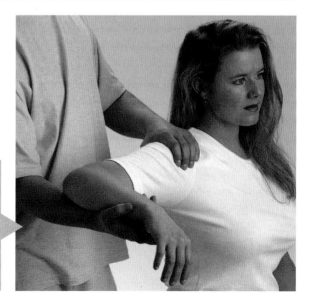

15 SQUEEZING AND KNEADING THE UPPER ARM

Repeat step 5 using your left hand, working along the length of the arm firmly and gently, but this time with a forward-pushing action.

16 PRESSING QI-POINTS

Repeat step 3, pressing and kneading **SJ 14** and **LI 15**, but this time with the thumb pressing into **SJ 14** and the middle finger pressing **LI 15**. From the back, knead **SI 10**, **SI 11**, **SI 12**, **SI 13**, **SI 14** and **SI 15** (see page 39).

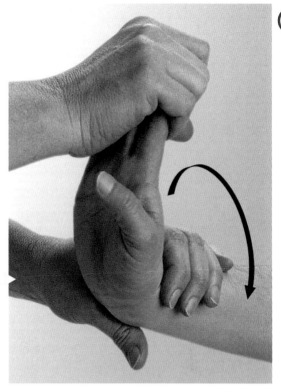

17 ROTATING WRIST, FINGERS AND THUMB

With your left hand, grasp your partner's forearm just above the wrist, and with your right hand grasp the fingers. Rotate the hand on the wrist in both directions for several minutes.

This technique promotes qi-flow through the six meridians passing through the wrist.

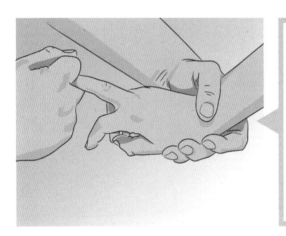

18 PULLING THE FINGERS

Supporting the wrist with your left hand, vigorously rotate each of the fingers and thumb in turn. Pull each one firmly by sliding it between your crooked index and second fingers to produce a strong flick. Finally, roll each finger and thumb in turn firmly between your palms.

Each finger stretch opens the joints to prevent arthritis and stimulates all the six meridians that begin or end in the fingers (see pages 38–41 and 50–51).

19 HAND STRETCH

With your partner's palm facing upwards, grip the sides of the hand between your fingers and the heel of your thumb. Stretch the hand sideways and outwards several times. In this position, press and knead **P 8**, **P 7**, **P 6**, **H 7**, **LU 9** and **LU 10**.

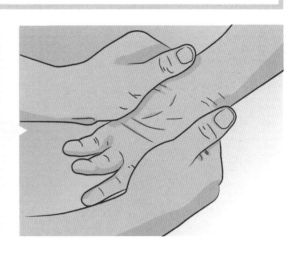

20 ROTATING THE ARM

Stand behind your partner's right shoulder. With your left hand, grasp the top of the shoulder, pressing **SJ 14** and **LI 15**. Support the right arm with your right hand under the elbow. Gently rotate the arm backwards with small movements, gradually increasing the range of movement. Don't attempt full rotation if there is any pain. Rotate the arm at least three times against the pressure of your thumb on **SJ 14**. Repeat in the opposite direction, pressing into **LI 15**.

The rotation and pressure on qi-points improves joint mobility and eases pain.

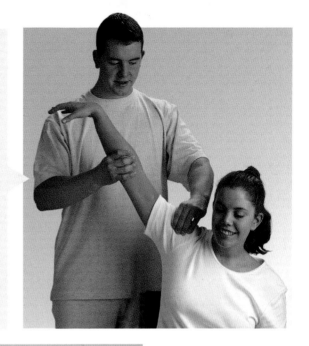

REPEAT STEPS 1–20 FROM PAGES 90–96, THIS TIME ON THE LEFT SIDE OF THE BODY.

When you have finished both arms and shoulders, return to the neck and shoulders and repeat any of the steps to leave your partner feeling totally relaxed.

The routines described so far are for balancing the qi in the upper body and will leave your partner invigorated, relaxed and sparkling.

21 LEVERED UPPER BACK STRETCH

Your partner raises their arms and, with fingers interlocked, turns the palms upwards above the head. Stand behind your partner and place the palm of your left hand in the middle of the upper back (over thoracic vertebrae five and six). Grasp the joined hands with your right hand and gently pull them towards you while pushing forwards with your left hand. Be very sensitive and don't pull the hands back further than is comfortable. Slightly reposition your left hand and repeat five times.

Caution: don't attempt this or step 22 with an elderly or frail partner.

This shoulder manipulation is an effective way of stretching the pectoral and deltoid muscles. It improves mobility of the shoulder joints.

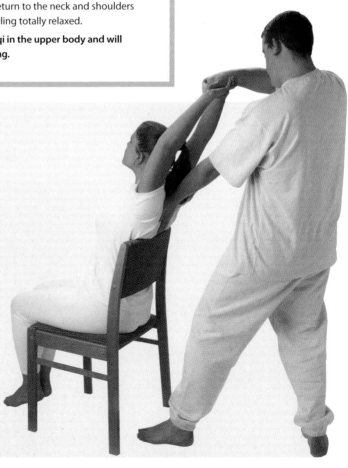

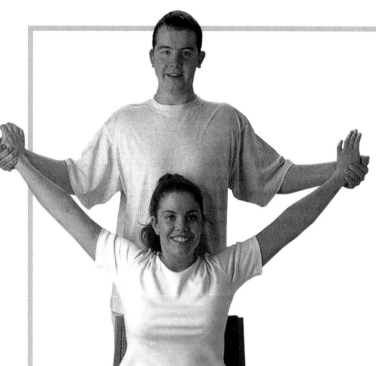

22 ARM AND SHOULDER STRETCH

Standing behind your partner, with their arms raised above the head, grasp each arm around the base of the thumb. Gently twist both arms outwards to create a slight stretch. Draw the arms apart, slowly and carefully, and back until you feel resistance. Hold the position for at least thirty seconds and repeat several times.

Like step 21, this manipulation gives a big stretch to the front of the shoulders and the chest.

23 FIRM PALMAR KNEAD WITH PUSHING AND PUMMELLING ON THE BACK

Your partner sits, with legs straight, on the edge of the chair, leaning forwards to touch the legs as far down as possible. Push firmly down the spine on the bladder meridian to the lumbar region with the heel of your hand. Repeat this several times on both sides of the spine and then repeat down the du meridian. Pummel with alternating hands down both sides of the spine (but not on the spine).

Relaxes the back and invigorates your partner by removing stagnation in the bladder and du meridians. It's a good way to finish the sitting routine.

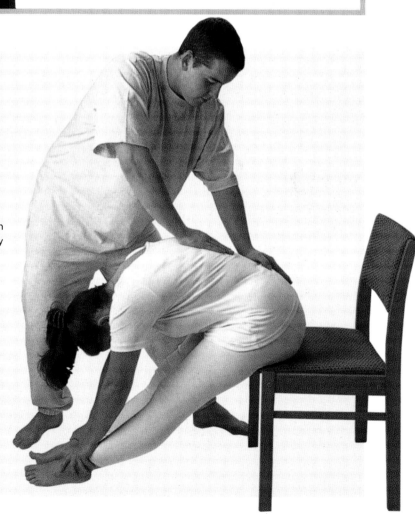

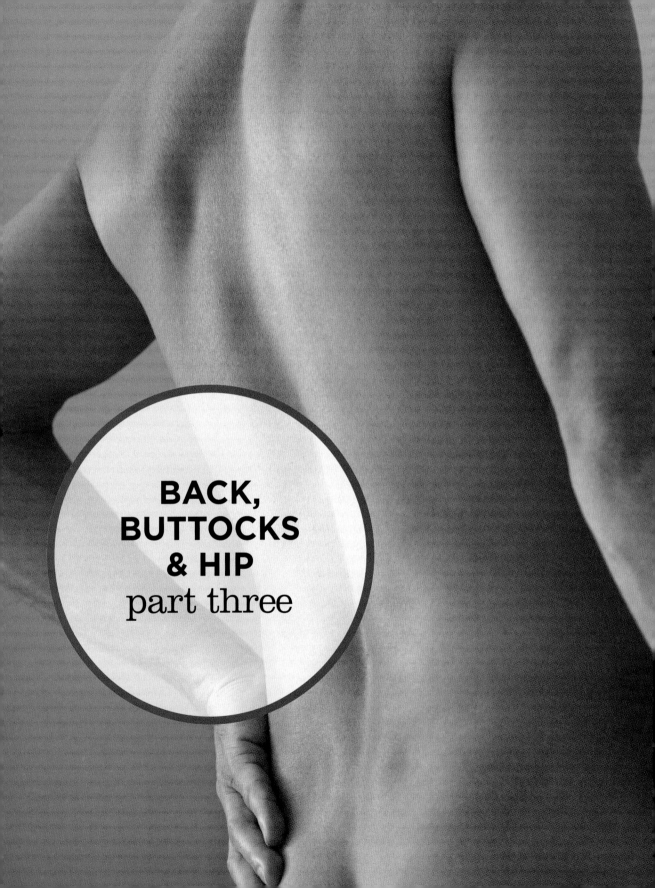

BACK, BUTTOCKS & HIP
part three

Main qi-points

The diagram below shows the qi-points that can be massaged when Tui Na is applied to the back, buttocks and hips. Back shu qi-points are found on the bladder meridian (blue). The hip qi-points are on the gall bladder meridian (green). The distance from the centre of the spine to the inner margins of the scapula is 3 cun. The back shu qi-points are located 1.5 cun from the midline.

BACK SHU POINTS –
balance their related organs

BL 11 Bone
BL 12 Wind gate
BL 13 Lung
BL 14 Pericardium
BL 15 Heart
BL 16 Du
BL 17 Blood
BL 18 Liver
BL 19 Gall bladder
BL 20 Spleen
BL 21 Stomach
BL 22 Sanjiao
BL 23 Kidney
BL 24 Sea of qi
BL 25 Large intestine
BL 26 Gate of yuan qi
BL 27 Bladder
BL 28 Small intestine
BL 29 Back muscle
BL 30 White ring
BL 31 Upper crevice
BL 32 Second crevice
BL 33 Middle crevice
BL 34 Lower crevice

LOWER BACK POINT

BL 54 Outer bladder meridian

HIP POINTS

GB 29
GB 30

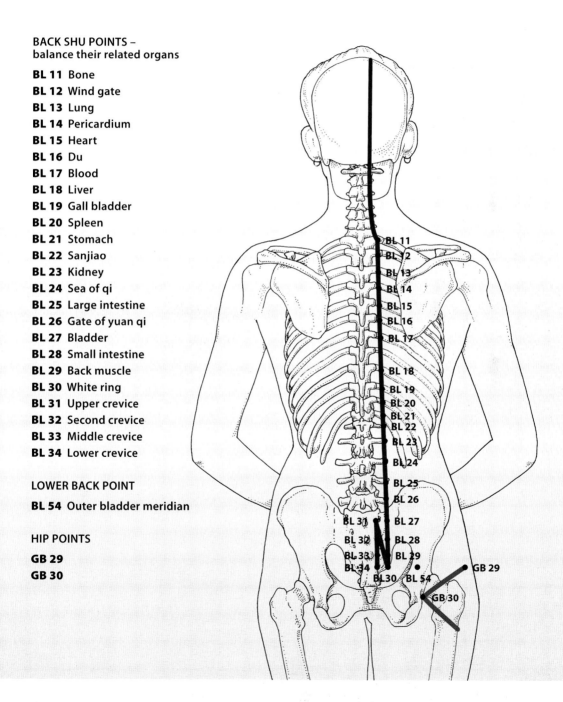

Your partner lies face down, with arms by the sides. This part of the routine stimulates the shu points of the bladder meridian for overall well-being (see page 26), reduces tension and pain in the whole back and eases sciatica. You will be working on the left side first, followed by the right.

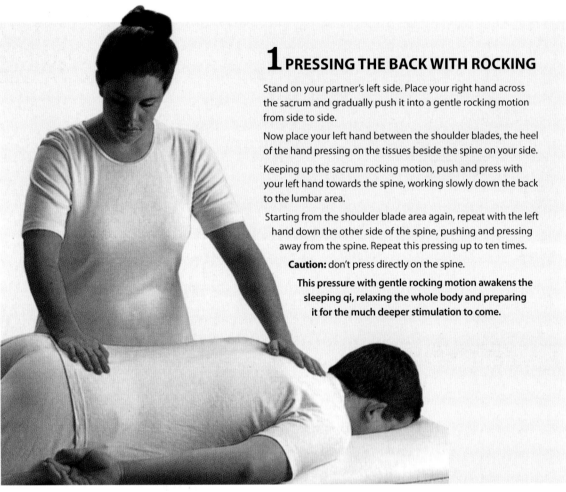

1 PRESSING THE BACK WITH ROCKING

Stand on your partner's left side. Place your right hand across the sacrum and gradually push it into a gentle rocking motion from side to side.

Now place your left hand between the shoulder blades, the heel of the hand pressing on the tissues beside the spine on your side.

Keeping up the sacrum rocking motion, push and press with your left hand towards the spine, working slowly down the back to the lumbar area.

Starting from the shoulder blade area again, repeat with the left hand down the other side of the spine, pushing and pressing away from the spine. Repeat this pressing up to ten times.

Caution: don't press directly on the spine.

This pressure with gentle rocking motion awakens the sleeping qi, relaxing the whole body and preparing it for the much deeper stimulation to come.

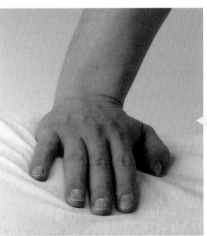

2 SINGLE HAND KNEADING ON THE BACK

Place the heel of one hand with the fingers relaxed on your partner's upper back between the spine and the left shoulder blade, level with **BL 13**. Pressure is focused through the heel, not the palm or fingers. Vigorously knead in a small circle in one place about twenty times. Knead progressively down the back to the sacrum along the bladder meridian. Repeat several times.

Single kneading promotes the qi-flow in the bladder meridian, which stimulates the internal organs.

3 SINGLE HEEL OF HAND KNEADING ON THE BACK

Repeat step 2 using just the heel of the hand to knead smoothly to and fro in one place before moving down the back along the bladder meridian.

This very focused kneading moves the underlying tissues to release muscle tension in the back.

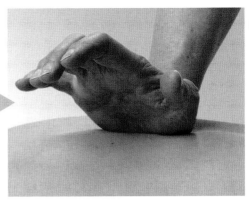

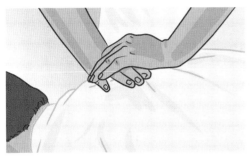

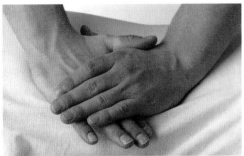

4 DOUBLE HAND KNEADING ON THE BACK

Place the heels of both hands side by side between the spine and the left shoulder blade, level with **BL 13**. Cross the fingers of the left hand over those of the right. With a circular motion, knead vigorously in one place about twenty times. This kneading creates side-to-side movement in the whole body. Work in this way down the back to the sacrum. Repeat several times.

Double kneading on the back shu qi-points will powerfully stimulate the organs to which they are energetically linked.

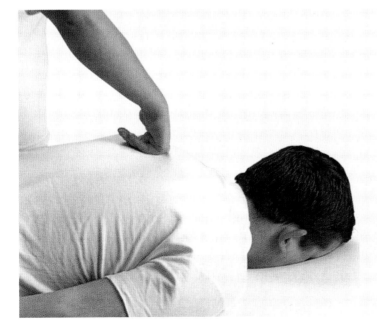

5 ROLLING DOWN THE BACK

Stand beside your partner, facing towards the head. Place your right hand between the spine and left shoulder blade, with your little finger over the spine. Start at **BL 13** level. Use the single rolling technique down the left of the spine to the sacrum as you step backwards. Lift your hand rather than sliding it between positions and roll firmly about thirty times in each position.

Single rolling stimulates the inner bladder meridian. The rhythm aids relaxation and softens knotted muscles.

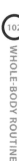

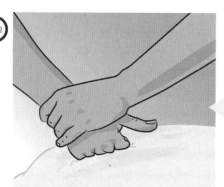

6 ROLLING TOWARDS THE SPINE

Facing your partner, use the double rolling technique, progressing from the top of the back down to the lumbar area. With firm pressure, place your second finger joints on the inner bladder meridian and roll towards the spine, at least twenty times at each position. During each roll, your knuckles will be just above the spinous processes.

The combined effects of these rolling techniques on the bladder meridian release tension throughout the back.

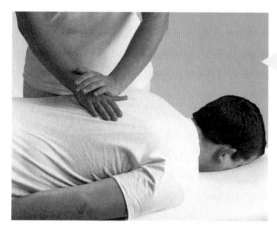

7 KNEAD BY PLUCKING ALONG THE SPINE

Place your thumb on the inner bladder meridian. Knead by plucking towards the spine, following the same path as you do in step 4. Be guided by your partner in how much pressure to use, increasing the pressure on the lower back.

This series of techniques increases qi-flow through the back and all the organs affected by the bladder meridian.

8 KNEADING QI-POINTS

With the middle finger and thumb of the left hand on top of the middle finger and thumb of the right hand, knead by pressing and pushing forwards and backwards on all the bladder meridian qi-points in turn, from **BL 11** to **BL 23**, on both sides of the spine simultaneously.

From **BL 23**, gradually increase the pressure and the size of movement, setting up a body rocking action from the arm. Repeat on **BL 24**, **BL 25** and **BL 26**. Your partner may well feel 'pleasurable pain' with this technique. Knead each point for two minutes.

Kneading the bladder meridian shu points balances the organs (see page 99) for optimum function. BL 23–26 have a key role in maintaining a healthy, pain-free lower back and can treat slipped lumbar discs if massaged daily.

Thumb kneading BL 27–30 maintains flexibility of the sacroiliac joint. Kneading BL 31–34 improves qi-flow to the sacrum. To powerfully strengthen the kidney energies knead BL 23 and GB 25, the kidney mu point.

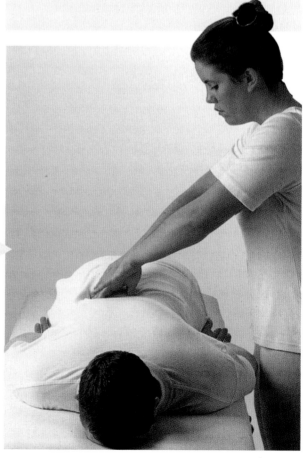

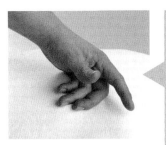

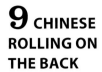

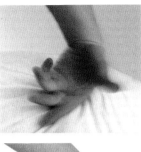

9 CHINESE ROLLING ON THE BACK

With either hand or alternating hands, use the Chinese rolling technique to roll quickly and firmly over the whole back.

This relaxing technique contrasts with the previous more penetrating ones. Any residual tension is dispersed, leaving your partner feeling relaxed and ready for the next phase.

10 FOREARM KNEADING ON THE BACK

Use the upper third of the forearms together across the middle of the back. Move your arms apart as you knead over the entire back. Leaning in with your body weight, apply outward pressure to achieve lengthwise and diagonal stretches. Repeat on the other side.

This technique gently stretches the back, helping to relax muscles.

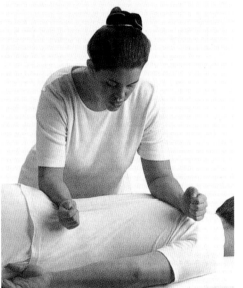

11 CHAFING THE BACK

Standing on your partner's left, chafe rapidly along each side of the spine in turn. Use long, firm strokes, at least twenty strokes on each side. Then use two-hand chafing across the sacrum, making at least fifty very rapid, short to and fro strokes. This can also be done on a bare back, using a little massage oil on the skin.

Chafing stimulates the bladder meridian and the kidneys. On the sacrum it can bring warmth down to the feet, because it moves qi rapidly through the bladder meridian to the legs.

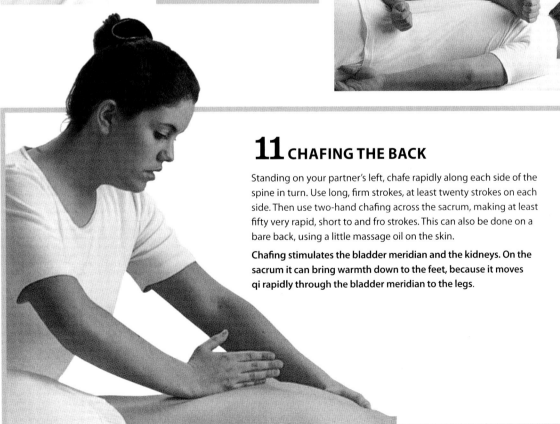

12 PERCUSSION ON THE BACK AND BUTTOCKS

Stand on your partner's left and use cupping over the buttocks and sacrum. Then cup up the spine with the hand lengthways along it (see page 71). Use some force over the buttocks and sacrum but go gently along the spine. Repeat several times. Then, still standing on your partner's left, pummel quickly, lightly and rhythmically several times down both sides of the spine, but not on the spine itself. Finish with hacking on all areas of soft tissue on the back.

These percussive techniques are tremendously stimulating and promote qi and blood circulation.

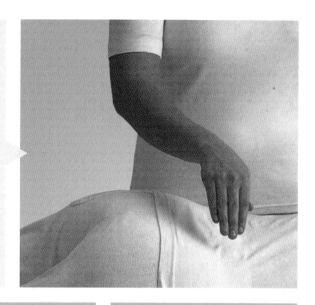

REPEAT STEPS 1–12 ON YOUR PARTNER'S RIGHT SIDE

In step 3, face your partner's feet and not the head when rolling down the side of the spine, to ensure that you use your stronger right hand.

AFTER REPEATING STEPS

1–12 on your partner's right side, you can do steps 13 and 14 to finish off the back routine.

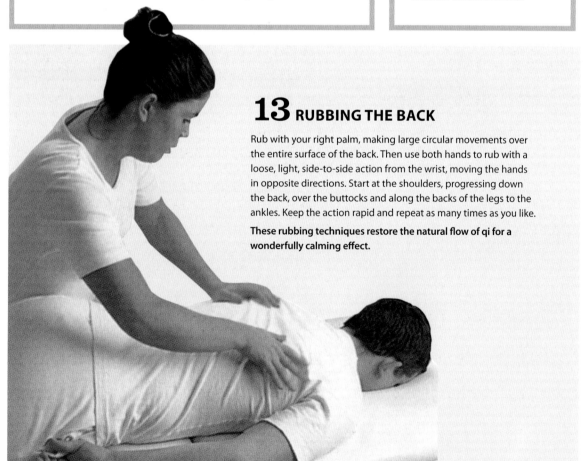

13 RUBBING THE BACK

Rub with your right palm, making large circular movements over the entire surface of the back. Then use both hands to rub with a loose, light, side-to-side action from the wrist, moving the hands in opposite directions. Start at the shoulders, progressing down the back, over the buttocks and along the backs of the legs to the ankles. Keep the action rapid and repeat as many times as you like.

These rubbing techniques restore the natural flow of qi for a wonderfully calming effect.

14 PALMAR KNEAD WITH PUSHING THE BACK AND LEGS

Standing on your partner's left side, place your right hand along the spine at the base of the neck, fingers pointing towards the feet. Push firmly and deeply, down the du meridian to the sacrum. Then start at shoulder level and push forcefully down each side of the spine on the bladder meridian over the buttocks, and down each leg. On each ankle, squeeze and knead **BL 60** (see page 57) and **K 3** (see page 54).

Pushing in this way assists the flow of qi along the du and bladder meridians.

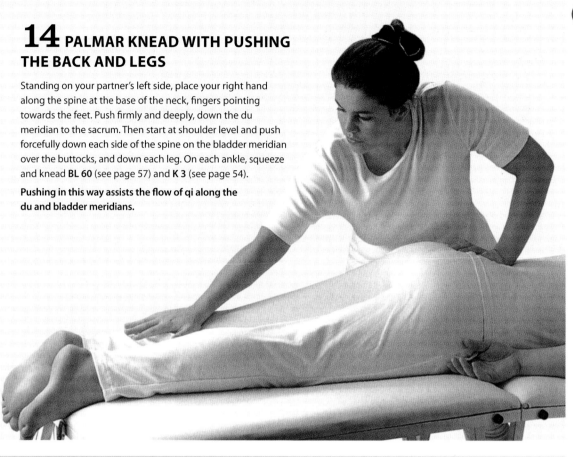

MANIPULATION TECHNIQUES FOR THE SHOULDER

These are not done as part of the basic routine but are useful if your partner has specific shoulder tension or pain. See page 72 under 'Joint manipulation techniques'.

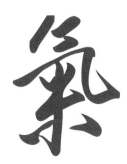

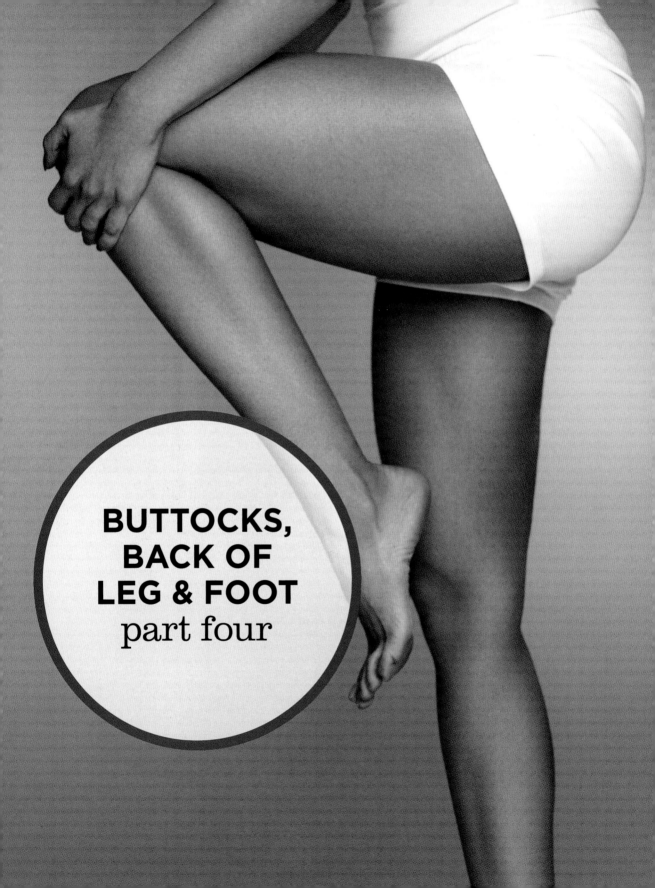

BUTTOCKS, BACK OF LEG & FOOT
part four

Main qi-points

The diagram below shows the qi-points that can be massaged when Tui Na is applied to the leg and foot. These are found on the following meridians: bladder and kidney (blue), gall bladder (green) and spleen and stomach (yellow).

XIYAN – extra point

Located in the medial knee eye (ST 35 is in the lateral knee eye). Treats knee pain.

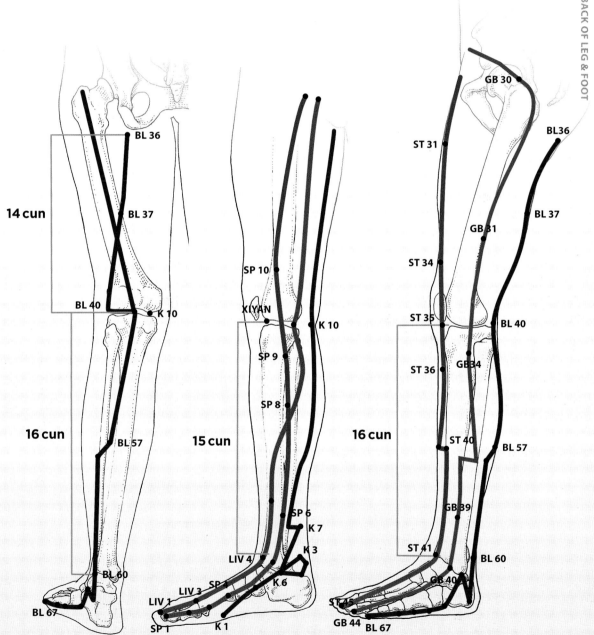

Carry out steps 1–10 on one leg first, then repeat the same steps on the other leg.

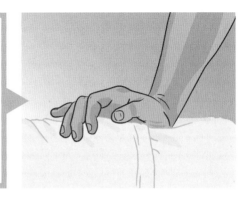

1 KNEADING THE BUTTOCKS

Start using single heel of hand kneading on the right buttock muscles. Move the heel of the hand to and fro, or in a circle for several minutes, focusing on **BL 54** (see pages 57 and 99) and **GB 30**. You can alternate with crossed double heel of palm kneading (see page 63).

Kneading the lumbar region and buttocks relieves chronic lower back pain and improves hip mobility.

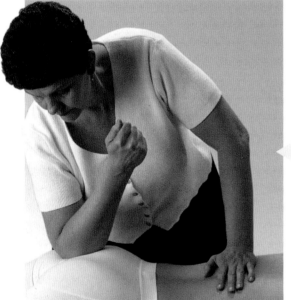

2 ELBOW KNEADING BUTTOCKS

Elbow knead over the whole area to relax the muscles. Press and knead **GB 30** and **BL 54** with the thumbs, and then with the elbow, making small circular movements. Lean in gradually with your body weight to give more pressure (but take care when doing this).

GB 30 and BL 54 are 'gateway points' through which qi flows between the spine and the legs. This qi-generating massage sequence is vital for lower back and hip joint flexibility and is a wonderful help for sciatica sufferers.

3 FOREARM KNEADING THE BUTTOCKS

For less penetrating pressure, use the upper third of the forearm instead of the tip of the elbow. Move your forearm with a firm kneading and pushing motion to achieve the best effect.

Relaxes the buttocks and improves hip mobility.

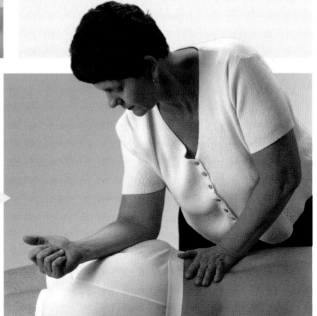

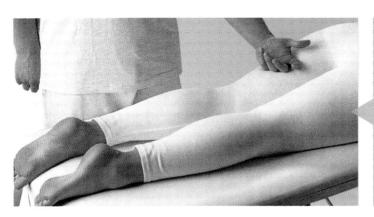

4 ROLLING THE LEG

With your partner lying face down, use Chinese or single rolling on the leg nearer to you. Work on the bladder meridian from the base of the buttock down to the ankle. Repeat at least twice.

5 KNEADING THE LEG

Knead deeply across the leg with the heel of one hand, starting just below the buttocks and working down to the ankle. Repeat the kneading, using both hands.

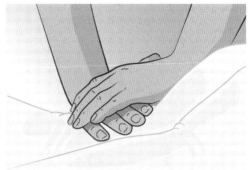

6 KNEADING AND SQUEEZING THE LEG

With your thumbs on one side of the leg and fingers on the other, use both hands side by side with a kneading, squeezing and lifting action down the leg on the bladder and gall bladder meridians to the ankle. Repeat several times.

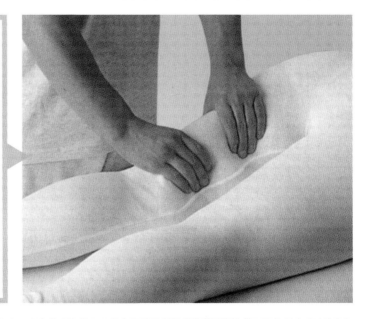

7 PRESSING AND KNEADING QI-POINTS ON THE BACK OF THE LEG

Press deeply with the elbow, using a rotary kneading action, into **BL 36** and **BL 37**, and with the thumb into **BL 40**, **K 10** and **BL 57**. Knead **BL 60** and **K 3** together with middle finger and thumb.

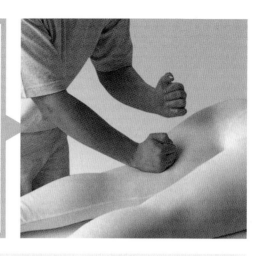

8 PERCUSSION ON THE LEGS

Using alternating pummelling work, from the buttocks down the middle of the back of the legs on the bladder meridian. Repeat several times. You can also use one-handed cupping or hacking with two hands.

These treatments leave the legs feeling wonderfully light. They relax tense muscles and can relieve sciatica and lower back pain.

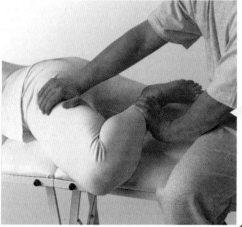

9 LEG IN FROG POSITION

Lifting the foot, slide the knee out to the side with your other hand. Let the foot rest across the back of the other leg. Strong, whole-hand kneading with a squeeze down the flexed leg on the gall bladder meridian moves the underlying tissues to clear stagnation. Rolling and percussion stimulate movement of qi. Press and knead **GB 30, GB 31, GB 34, GB 39** and **GB 40.**

Tui Na in this position relieves sciatic pain. GB 34 relieves muscle and tendon problems and GB 39 strengthens the bones.

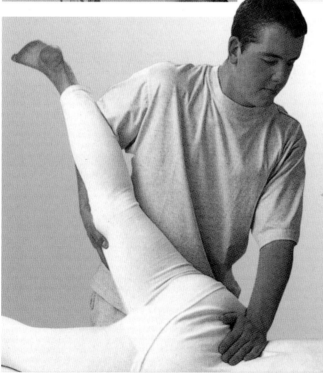

10 HIP ROTATION, AND LEG LIFT WITH LUMBAR PRESS MANIPULATION

Place one hand over **BL 25** (see page 56) on the side of the spine nearest you. Applying pressure to the lumbar area, lift the straight leg, supporting it just above the knee against your forearm. Raise the leg until you feel resistance, hold for a minute and then rotate it in small circles.

Aligns the hips, pelvis and lower back. Relieves lower back pain.

11 LUMBAR PRESS WITH FLEXED LEGS MANIPULATION

Place the heel of your hand across the lumbar area on **BL 25** (see page 56). Press deeply, while carefully and slowly pushing your partner's feet towards the buttocks with your other hand. Hold this for about a minute and repeat several times.

This manipulation treats lower back and sacroiliac pain.

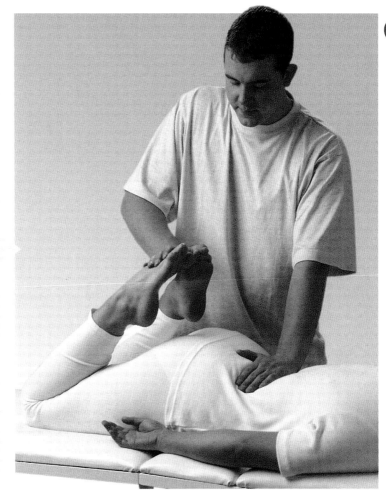

REPEAT STEPS 1–11 ON THE OTHER SIDE OF THE BODY, then follow steps 12–17 on one foot before repeating on the other foot.

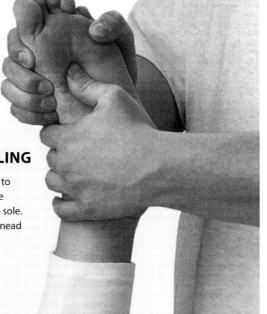

12 THUMB KNEADING AND PUMMELLING

With your partner lying face down, lift the lower leg nearest to you to expose the sole of the foot. Supporting the top of the foot with one hand, use the thumb of the other hand to knead deeply all over the sole. Then pummel using the edge of your lightly clenched fist. Thumb knead **K 1** (see page 54).

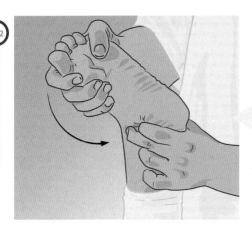

13 FOOT ROTATION

Grasp around the back of the ankle, pressing into **GB 40** and **LIV 4**. Holding the foot with your other hand, rotate it several times in both directions.

This stimulates qi-flow through the six meridians of the foot. Pressing GB 40 and LIV 4 strengthens the ankle.

14 HACKING THE ACHILLES TENDON

Support the front of the foot, pressing down on the toes to stretch the Achilles tendon. Slightly spread the fingers of the other hand and hack the tendon with the side of your hand.

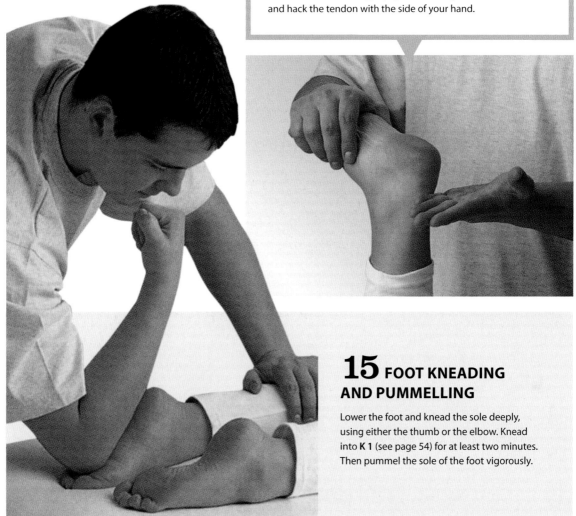

15 FOOT KNEADING AND PUMMELLING

Lower the foot and knead the sole deeply, using either the thumb or the elbow. Knead into **K 1** (see page 54) for at least two minutes. Then pummel the sole of the foot vigorously.

16 CHAFING THE SOLE

Holding the lower leg, chafe vigorously on the sole of the foot, following a diagonal line over **K 1** and over the arch of the foot. Chafe for two minutes.

K 1 brings the qi downwards, giving a wonderfully grounded feeling and improved sleep.

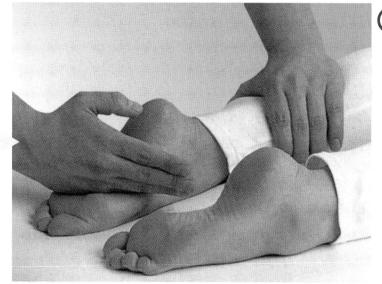

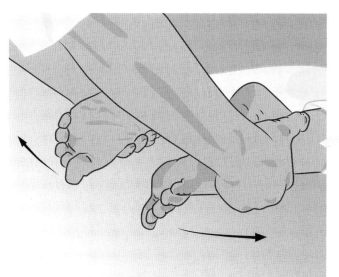

17 LATERAL LEG SWING

Grasp both feet under the ankles and lift them a little. Lean backwards, pulling the legs gently, and then swing them together from side to side creating a gentle rock on the hips and spine. Swing for several minutes.

This manipulation loosens the hip joints and relaxes the spinal muscles.

REPEAT STEPS 12–17 ON THE OTHER SIDE.

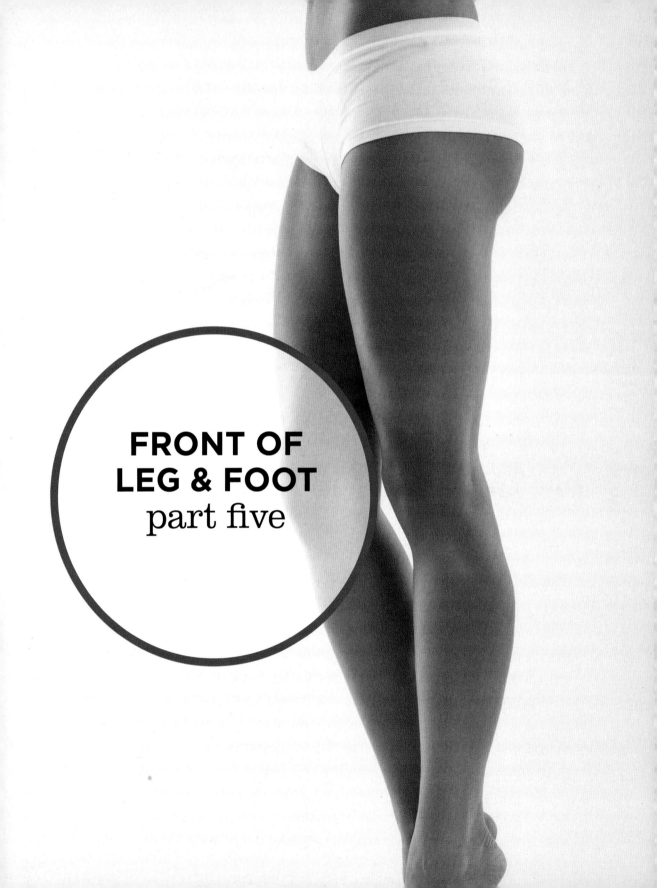

FRONT OF LEG & FOOT
part five

Main qi-points

The diagram below shows the qi-points that can be massaged when Tui Na is applied to the leg and foot. These are found on the following meridians: stomach (yellow), liver (green), kidney (blue) and spleen (yellow).

XIYAN – extra point

Located in the medial knee eye (ST 35 is in the lateral knee eye). Treats knee pain.

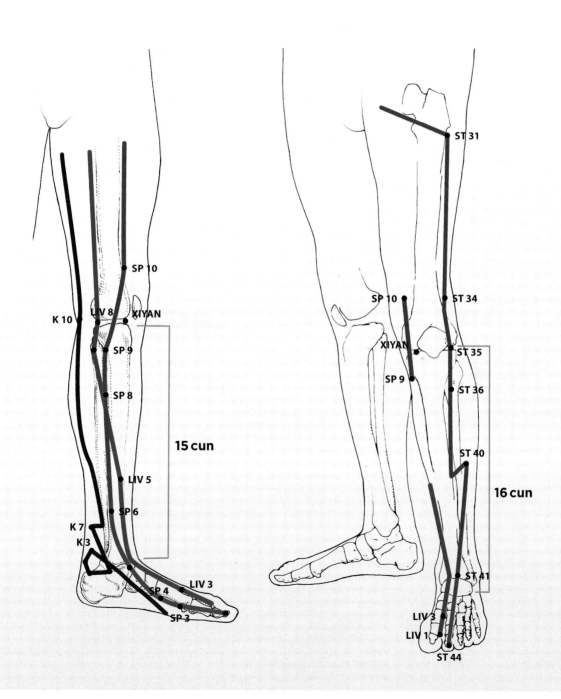

1 FRONT OF THE LEG

With your partner lying on their back, repeat steps
4, 5, 6 and 8 from Part Four (see pages 100–1),
carrying out rolling, kneading, squeezing (see right)
and percussion on the stomach and gall bladder
meridians. Press and knead **ST 31, ST 34** and **SP 10**
together, **ST 36, ST 40** and **GB 29, GB 31** and **GB 34**
(see pages 34 and 107).

**These techniques improve overall energy and
leg mobility.**

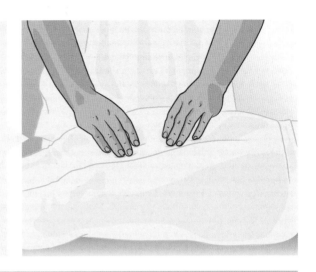

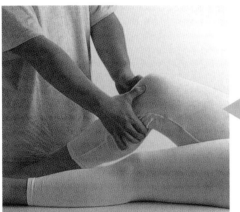

2 KNEE PRESSING WITH EXTENSION

Find the two depressions just below the kneecap. **ST 35** is in
the outside depression, while the inside one is an extra point
called xiyan, meaning 'knee eye'. Supporting the leg with your
fingers under it, press your thumb tips into each depression and
thumb knead deeply for several minutes. Still pressing the two
depressions, lift the knee up and pull the leg towards you.
Repeat this action several times.

ST 35 and xiyan maintain healthy knees and relieve knee pain.

3 INSIDE THE FLEXED LEG

Flex the leg out to the side, keeping the
foot tucked against the straight leg. Knead
with the heel of your hand, pushing over
the adductor muscles, and squeeze
along the entire inside length of the
flexed leg. Thumb press and knead
SP 10, SP 9, SP 8, SP 6 and **K 3.**

Caution: don't use **SP 6** during
pregnancy.

**Kneading the inner leg targets all
three yin meridians of the leg,
strengthening the spleen, kidney
and liver energies.**

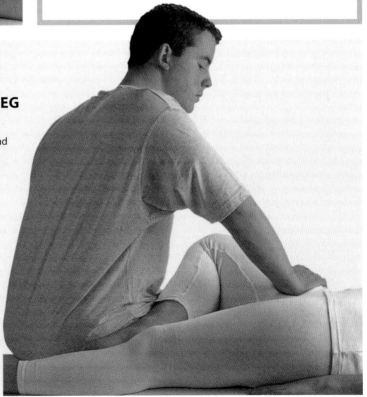

4 PRESSING THE CALF

Lift your partner's flexed leg and lock the foot by sitting on the toes. Place both hands behind the calf muscle and pull towards you progressively down the muscle on the bladder meridian. Knead **BL 57** (see page 57).

Pressure on the calf muscles relieves tension, spasm and sciatic pain.

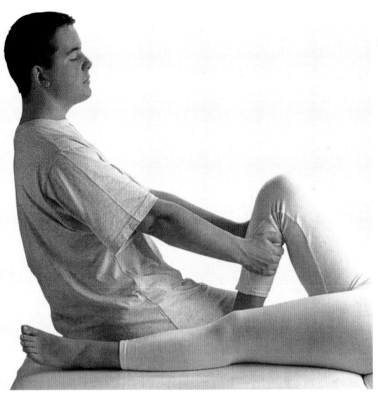

5 HIP ROTATION

Lift your partner's lower right leg over your right forearm and support the top of the knee with both hands, fingers interlocked. Rotate, making clockwise and anticlockwise circles. Start gently and gradually increase the size of the rotations as far as the joint allows. Another method is to support the heel with one hand and use the other hand on the knee to guide the rotation. This is a better method for more flexible people, who need larger rotations.

Frequent gentle rotations will Improve mobility of hip joints and ease arthritic hip pain, sciatica, lumbago and sacroiliac pain.

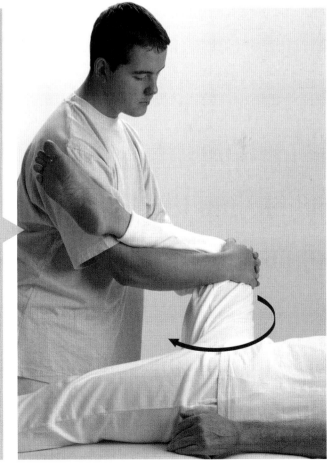

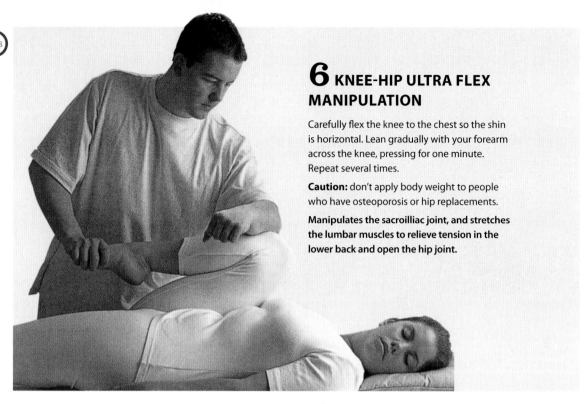

6 KNEE-HIP ULTRA FLEX MANIPULATION

Carefully flex the knee to the chest so the shin is horizontal. Lean gradually with your forearm across the knee, pressing for one minute. Repeat several times.

Caution: don't apply body weight to people who have osteoporosis or hip replacements.

Manipulates the sacroilliac joint, and stretches the lumbar muscles to relieve tension in the lower back and open the hip joint.

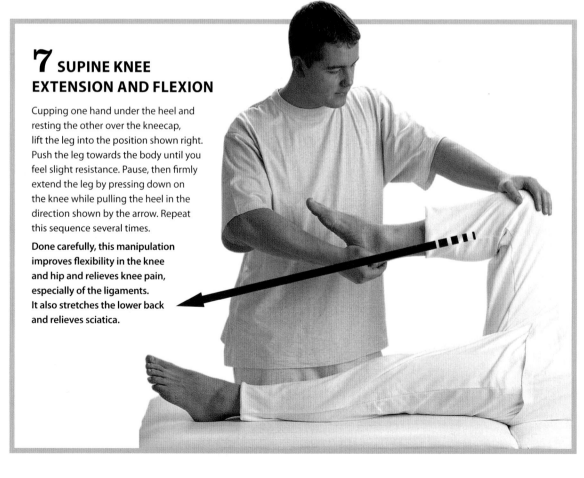

7 SUPINE KNEE EXTENSION AND FLEXION

Cupping one hand under the heel and resting the other over the kneecap, lift the leg into the position shown right. Push the leg towards the body until you feel slight resistance. Pause, then firmly extend the leg by pressing down on the knee while pulling the heel in the direction shown by the arrow. Repeat this sequence several times.

Done carefully, this manipulation improves flexibility in the knee and hip and relieves knee pain, especially of the ligaments. It also stretches the lower back and relieves sciatica.

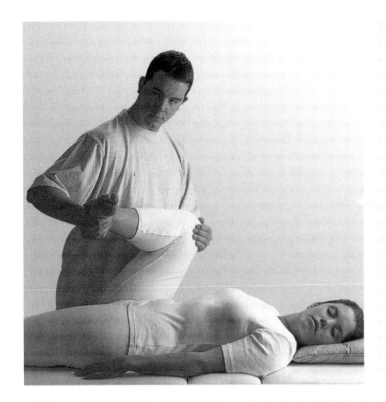

8 ZIG-ZAG HIP-KNEE ROCK

With the leg flexed so the shin is horizontal, hold the knee with one hand and the heel with the other. Carefully swing the knee outwards while swinging the heel towards the midline. Then reverse the movement to create fast, light to and fro actions, giving at least twenty swings in each direction.

Caution: don't use this technique on a knee replacement.

Releases connective tissue adhesions in the knee and hip to improve mobility.

9 LEG AND FOOT STRETCH

Place one hand under the heel with the sole against your forearm. With your other hand pressing down on the thigh just below the groin, lift the leg, keeping it straight. As you raise the leg, press your forearm against the foot to create a powerful ankle flexion. Relax and then repeat once or twice.

Stretching the bladder meridian improves tone in the calf muscles and hamstrings.

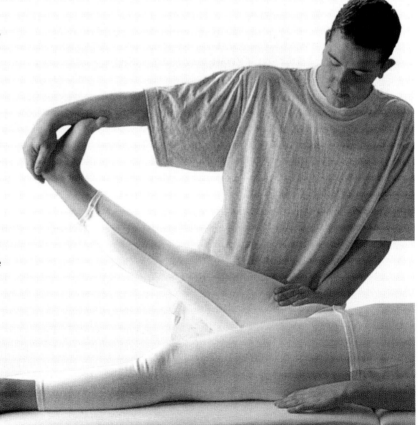

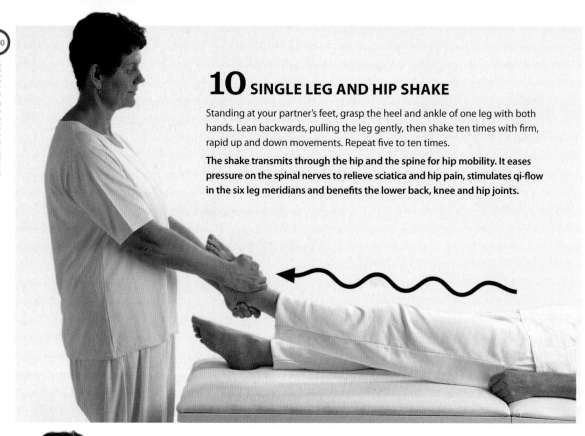

10 SINGLE LEG AND HIP SHAKE

Standing at your partner's feet, grasp the heel and ankle of one leg with both hands. Lean backwards, pulling the leg gently, then shake ten times with firm, rapid up and down movements. Repeat five to ten times.

The shake transmits through the hip and the spine for hip mobility. It eases pressure on the spinal nerves to relieve sciatica and hip pain, stimulates qi-flow in the six leg meridians and benefits the lower back, knee and hip joints.

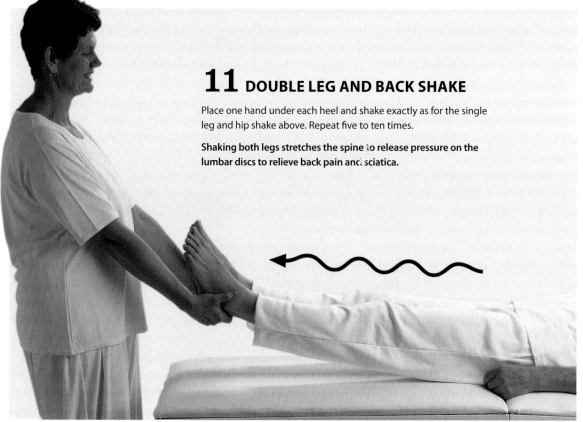

11 DOUBLE LEG AND BACK SHAKE

Place one hand under each heel and shake exactly as for the single leg and hip shake above. Repeat five to ten times.

Shaking both legs stretches the spine to release pressure on the lumbar discs to relieve back pain and sciatica.

12 FOOT ROTATION

Sit on the couch and lift your partner's nearest leg out and across so that the calf rests on your knee. Grasp the ankle with the supporting hand and rotate the foot with the other hand.

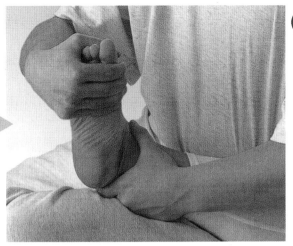

13 ANKLE ROTATION

With your partner lying on their back, raise the foot a little, supporting it with one hand under the lower leg just above the ankle. With your other hand, grip the toes and rotate the foot clockwise and anticlockwise.

This manipulation aids ankle mobility and treats a sprained ankle.

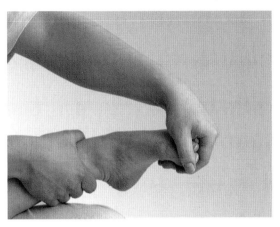

14 PULLING THE TOES

Grasp each toe in turn between your thumb and index finger. Rotate several times, and then pull vigorously.

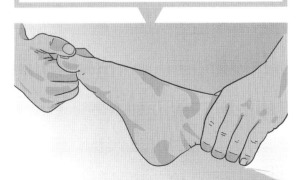

15 PRESSING AND KNEADING QI-POINTS

Use thumb pressing and kneading to stimulate **LIV 3, ST 44, SP 4, ST 41, K 3, K 6, GB 40** and **GB 43** (see pages 34 and 107 for GB points).

These qi-points on the foot have important local and distant effects. For example, GB 40 treats lateral ankle sprain and LIV 3 can relieve migraines.

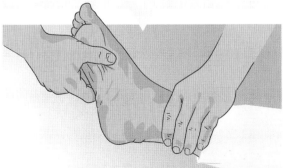

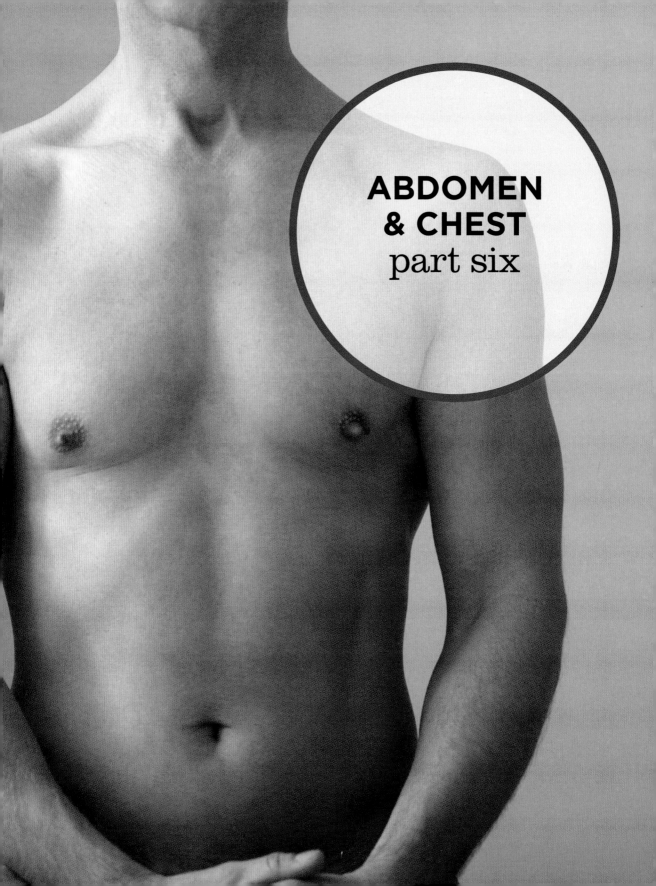

ABDOMEN
& CHEST
part six

Main qi-points

The diagram below shows the qi-points that can be massaged when Tui Na is applied to the abdomen and chest. These are found on the following meridians: lung (LU), ren (R), stomach and spleen (ST and SP), kidney (K), and liver and gall bladder (LIV and GB).

FRONT MU POINTS – strengthen their related organs

LU 1 Lung
R 17 Pericardium
R 14 Heart
R 12 Stomach
ST 25 Large intestine
R 5 Sanjiao
R 4 Small intestine
R 3 Bladder
LIV 13 Spleen
LIV 14 Liver
GB 24 Gall bladder
GB 25 Kidney (see page 35)

OTHER IMPORTANT POINTS

R 6 'Sea of qi' – tonifies qi
SP 15 Regulates spleen
ST 21 Regulates stomach
ST 29 Regulates reproduction
R 10 Regulates stomach
K 13 Regulates kidney
K 25, K 27 Regulates chest qi

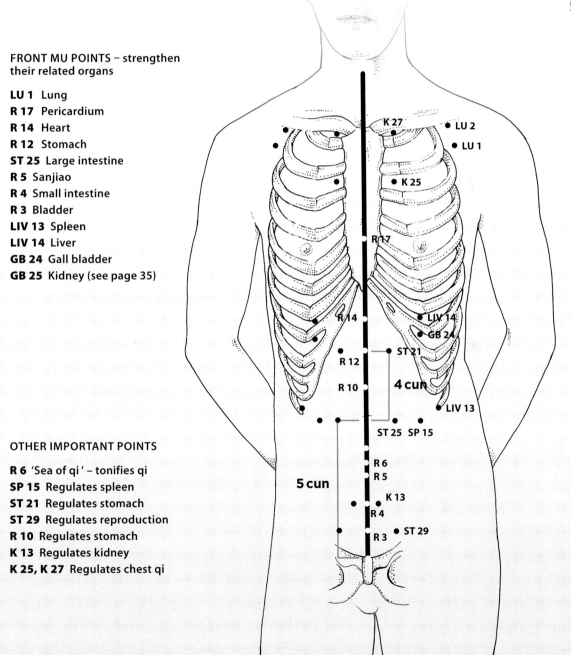

1 HEEL OF HAND KNEADING

Place the heel of your hand on your partner's abdomen on **R 4** – the area just above the pubic bone. Make clockwise kneading movements, gradually increasing the pressure. Using the square in step 2 (below) as a guide, heel knead in a clockwise direction progressively around the abdomen. Starting on **R 4**, knead around to **SP 15**, up to **R 12** and round, clockwise, to **SP 15**, and then back to **R 4**.

Caution: don't massage the abdomen during pregnancy.

Strengthens the stomach and spleen functions to assist digestion and ensure transformation of food and drink into qi. R 4 will tonify the spleen, liver and kidney functions.

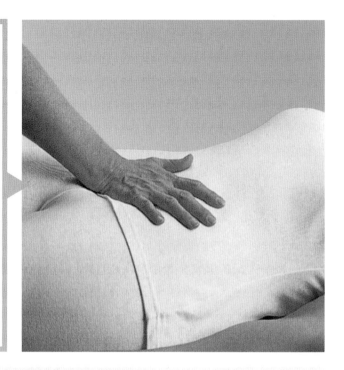

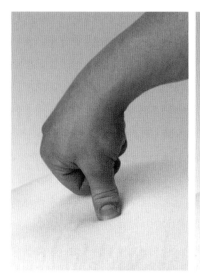

2 THUMB KNEADING ON ABDOMEN

Using the square (left) as a guide, and with both thumbs side by side, thumb knead the abdomen, starting on **R 4**. Progress up the right side to **SP 15** and then to **R 12**, always kneading towards the navel. Repeat this ten times.

Move to your partner's other side and repeat the kneading from **R 12** to **R 4** in the same way ten times. Adjust the pressure according to your partner's sensitivity.

These abdominal techniques can reduce the appetite if done daily for twenty minutes and also relieve constipation.

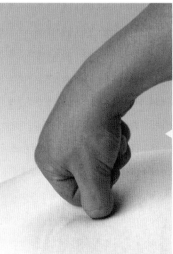

3 KNEADING QI-POINTS WITH THUMB ROCKING

Knead with thumb rock for several minutes on each of the qi-points **R 4**, **R 6** and **R 12**.

This technique boosts qi.

4 THUMB ROCKING THE REN MERIDIAN

Knead with thumb rock progressively down the ren meridian, starting with **R 17** and ending on **R 3**.

This stimulates the ren meridian to boost organ functions.

5 THUMB ROCKING THE STOMACH MERIDIANS

Knead with thumb rock progressively down each stomach meridian in turn, starting with **ST 21** and ending on **ST 29**. Also thumb knead **SP 15**. You can also do this with double thumb and finger kneading over each qi-point.

This technique boosts digestion and reproductive functions.

6 PALMAR KNEADING THE CHEST

Use the heel of the hand or the heel of the thumb to knead the entire chest. For a woman, don't knead the breast. Use the thumb to knead the intercostal muscles between the ribs.

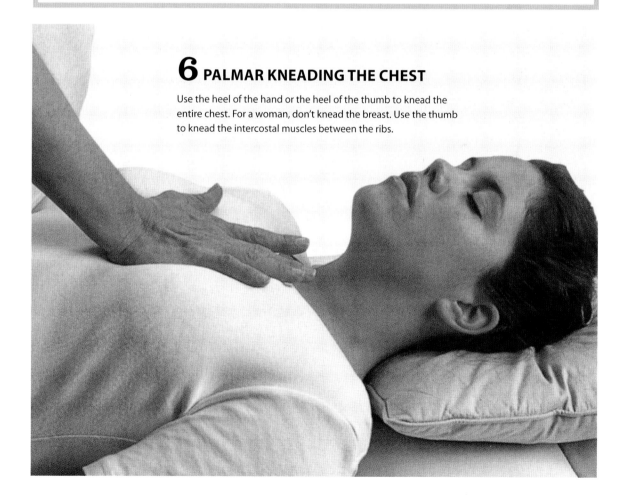

7 PRESSING AND KNEADING QI-POINTS

Thumb knead **R 17**, **R 14**, **LU 1**, **LU 2**, **K 25** and **K 27**.

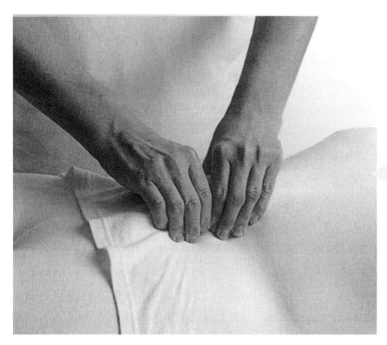

8 SQUEEZE, LIFT AND SHAKE

Squeeze with the fingers and thumbs of both hands as much excess, fatty abdominal tissue as you can comfortably hold. Lift and shake vigorously several times and then let go. For overweight partners, repeat anywhere on the abdomen for up to ten minutes.

Helps to break down abdominal fat by enhancing the circulation of blood and lymph through the adipose tissue.

9 INTERLOCKED HAND SQUEEZE AND KNEAD

With fingers interlocked, hand squeeze and knead firmly up and down the centre of the abdomen. Give each squeeze a circular kneading action with the heels of the hands. Repeat for two minutes.

Abdominal Tui Na can relieve irritable bowel syndrome by stimulating spleen and stomach function.

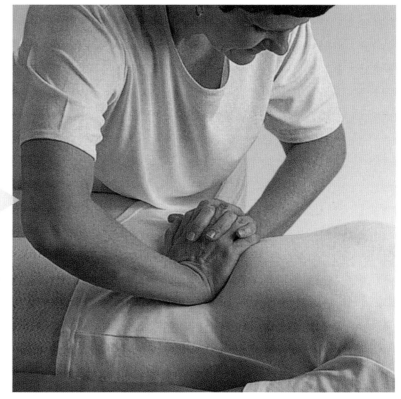

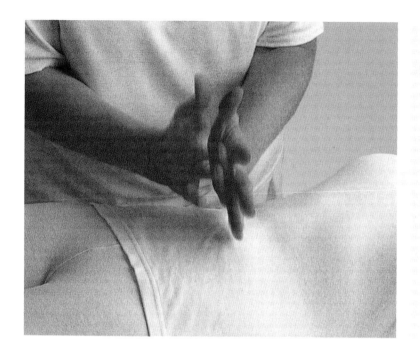

10 HACKING ON THE ABDOMEN

Using both hands separately, hack lightly over the entire abdominal area with the fingers loosely apart.

Boosts qi and blood flow in the abdomen.

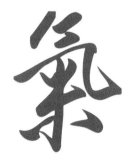

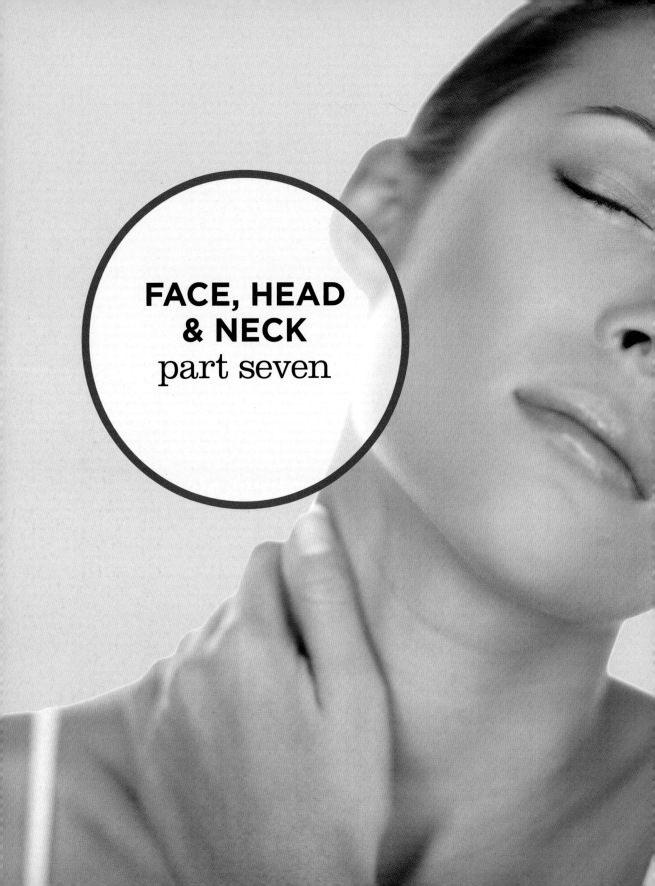

FACE, HEAD & NECK
part seven

Main qi-points

These are found on the following meridians: bladder (blue), small intestine (red), gall bladder (green), sanjiao (red), stomach (yellow), and du and ren (black).

YINTANG – extra point

Midway between the inner ends of the eyebrows. Treats insomnia and calms the mind.

TAIYANG – extra point

In a depression approximately 1 cun to the side of the outer corner of the eye and eyebrow. The point is calming, treats lateral headaches and eases head cold symptoms.

FOR A REFRESHING AND CALMING FACIAL MASSAGE:

Press and knead **BL 2** bilaterally with your middle fingers at least fifty times. Repeat on **SJ 23**, **GB 1**, **ST 1**, **GB 13**, **GB 14** and **taiyang** points for healthy eyes.
For good hearing, press and knead **SI 19**, **GB 2** and **SJ 17**.
For clear sinuses, press and knead **LI 20** and **ST 3**.
For healthy jaws, press and knead **ST 6**, **ST 7** and **DU 26**.

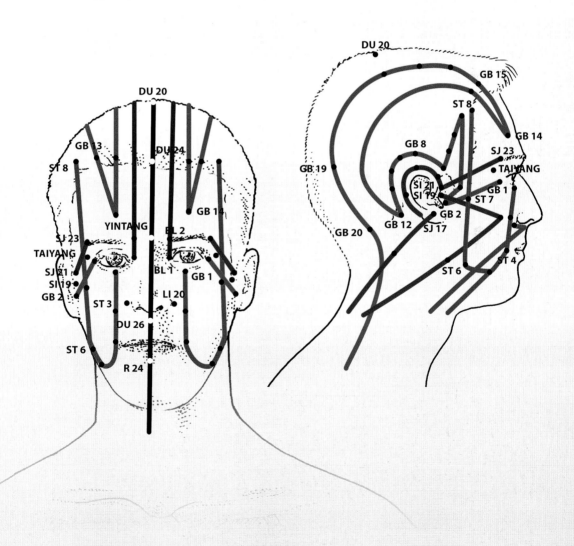

1 KNEADING

With your partner lying on their back, stand behind the head. Use the heels of both hands to knead firmly from the midline of the forehead over **GB 14** towards **taiyang** on the temples. Knead the **taiyang** points about twenty times and progressively knead the sides of the head to just above the ears, finishing on **GB 8**. Repeat twenty times.

Kneading GB 13, GB 14, taiyang and GB 8 clears and refreshes the head.

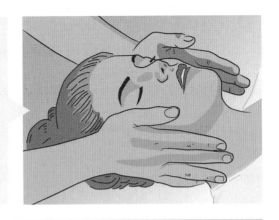

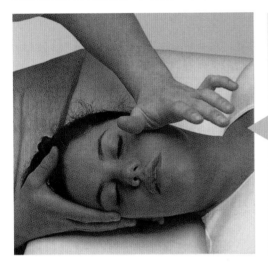

2 HEEL OF THE THUMB KNEADING THE FACE

Starting on the forehead, use the fleshy area (**LU 10** – see page 89) at the base of the thumb to vigorously knead across the forehead from one temple to the other, using a relaxed side-to-side rocking action. Repeat for several minutes. Then tilt the head to one side and knead down the cheek area, around the chin, then – tilting the head the other way – up the other cheek and around the forehead, to complete the cycle. Repeat several times.

This technique enhances blood and qi-flow to the skin with excellent cosmetic results.

3 THUMB KNEADING THE FACE

With quick, firm thumb strokes, push outwards from the midline of the forehead at **yintang** over the eyebrows to the **taiyang** points on the temples (see right). Repeat several times, moving your starting point from the eyebrows to the hairline on the du meridian.

Repeat this technique on the cheeks, starting from **ST 3**, just below the eyes, then from **LI 20**, **DU 26** and, finally, from **R 24**, moving progressively down the face with each stroke, always finishing on the **taiyang** points.

Improves blood flow in the skin, making the face glow.

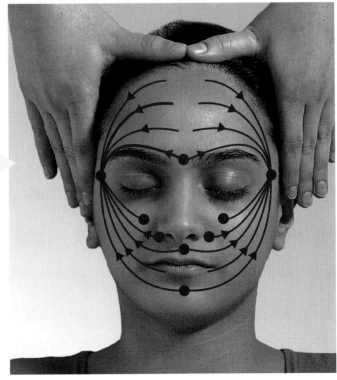

4 THUMB RUBBING THE FOREHEAD

From the **yintang** point between the eyebrows, use rapid, alternate thumb strokes, up the centre of the forehead.

5 THUMB ROCKING

Place the thumb pad on the **yintang** point, keeping your fingers straight. Moving the relaxed hand with side-to-side swinging movements, thumb rock for several minutes.

Yintang powerfully relaxes and calms the mind, leading to good sleep.

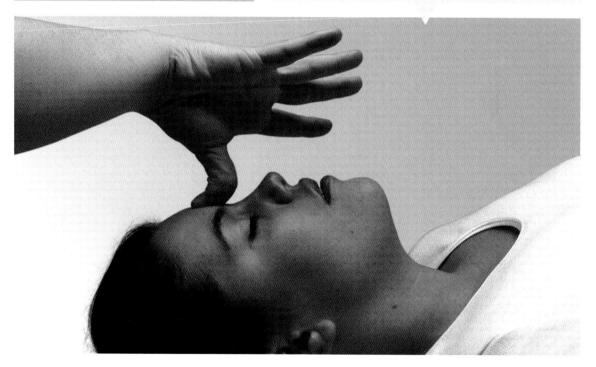

6 KNEADING THE SCALP

With the fingers of both hands, knead the entire scalp vigorously. Keep contact throughout and use small side-to-side or circular movements.

Boosts hair growth and stimulates the brain.

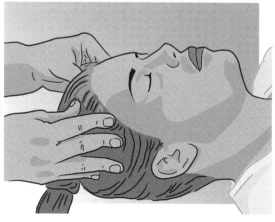

7 RUBBING THE HEAD

Starting with your left hand on the right side of your partner's head, rub to and fro around the outer edge of the ear along the gall bladder meridian with the tips of your fingers and thumb. The motion comes from a sideways rocking of the wrist. Repeat with your right hand on the left-hand side.

Rubbing over GB 8 will ease and prevent tension headaches.

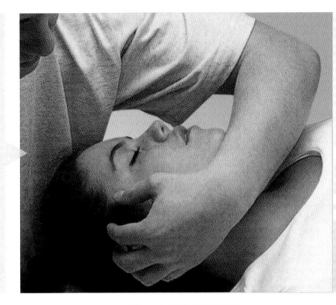

8 PRESSING SCALP MERIDIANS

With your thumbs one on top of the other, press from **yintang** to **DU 20**. Press firmly, repeating several times. Repeat on the bladder meridian, starting at **BL 2**, and again on the gall bladder meridian, starting from **GB 14**.

Pressing the du, bladder and gall bladder meridians stimulates the body's yang energies to clear and relax the mind.

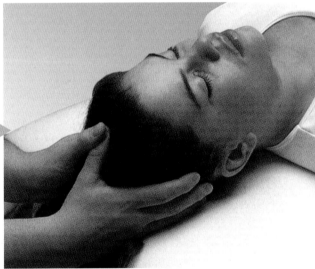

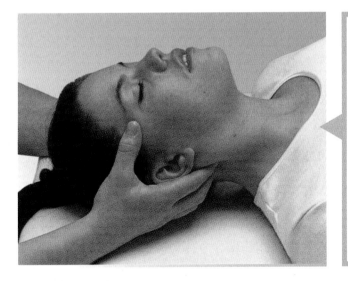

9 PULLING THE NECK

Slide your fingers under the neck to the occipital region of the skull. Knead both **GB 20** and **BL 10** (see page 56) firmly for several minutes. Hook the index and middle fingers into **GB 20** on both sides, lift and pull gently, holding the position for one minute.

Excellent treatment for headache and tense, painful neck muscles.

10 LIFTING THE NECK

Line up the fingers of both your hands under the
neck on either side of the spine on the bladder
meridian. With your fingertips, lift first one side
of the neck and then the other, so that the head
rocks from side to side. Repeat several times.

**This helps to relax tense neck muscles and
relieves a stiff neck.**

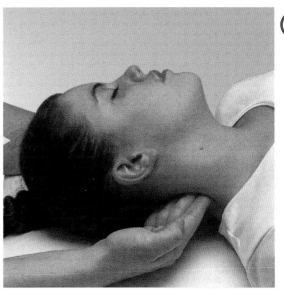

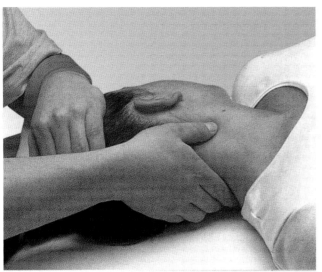

11 KNEADING THE NECK

Lift the head and turn it gently to one side.
Thumb knead along the band of muscle
from below the ear towards the collarbone.
Press and knead **GB 20** and **BL 10** (see
page 56). Repeat on the other side.

**Good for side neck pain, while GB 20
and BL 10 can treat all headaches.**

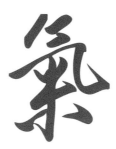

EVERYDAY
TUI NA

• • • • • • • • • • • • • • • • • • •

*Once you are familiar with the techniques described
in chapter 4, and have practised giving the whole-body
routine in chapter 5, you will be able to apply that
knowledge to relieve everyday symptoms
such as headaches and stiff shoulders. The Tui Na
in this chapter covers a range of treatments for
musculoskeletal conditions and common ailments
with their underlying causes and symptoms.
Before starting any Tui Na treatment, you should
check the cautions given on page 62.*

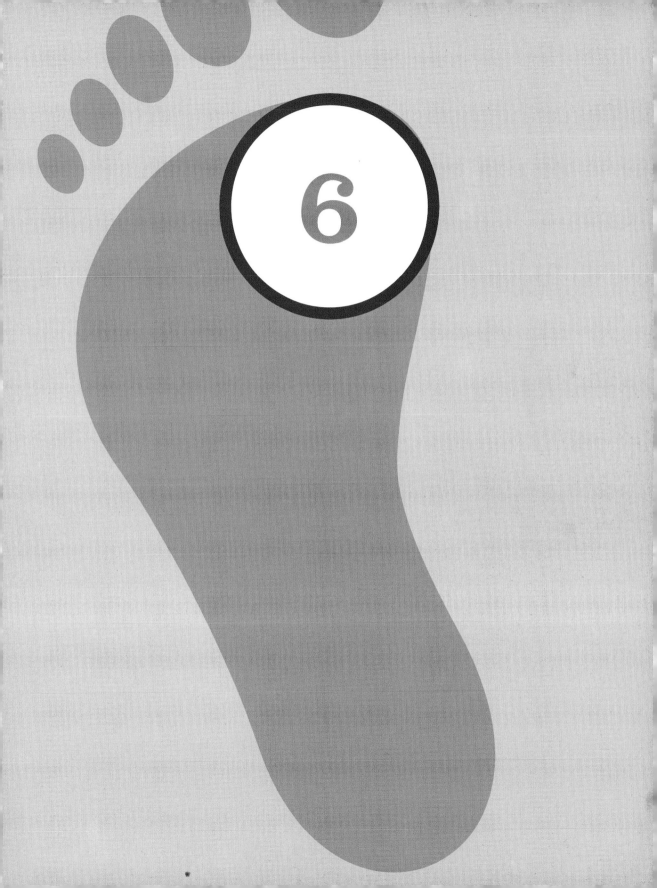

One of Tui Na's strengths is its ability to treat chronic and acute pain. Long-term, chronic, musculoskeletal pain may be caused by 'wear and tear' on the joints, often described as arthritis. Acute pain is usually caused by sports injuries or other traumas. Tui Na for chronic or acute musculoskeletal pain is presented on pages 138–43. Treatments for common ailments are presented on pages 143–6, arranged by ailment. These include everyday problems where you can use Tui Na safely to give relief from the ailment symptoms.

Tui Na is a valuable therapy for treating many of the problems associated with different life stages. Treatments particularly suitable for adolescents are described on page 147, and for the elderly on page 149. Three special techniques for babies and infants are given on pags 131. These promote health and strengthen the immune system. Tui Na for children under the age of five uses additional specialized finger and hand techniques not included in this book. The chapter ends with a daily self-help routine that will enable you to start every day with your qi-flow balanced and feeling full of sparkle and vitality.

UNDERLYING CAUSES OF PAIN

Traditional Chinese medicine regards all pain as the result of an imbalance in qi. Balancing qi-flow can reduce or even eliminate pain, even if the Western diagnosis is 'incurable'. Many everyday health problems are caused or exacerbated by stress, which can result from both emotional and physical causes. Common physical causes of tension include long periods sitting in a car or at a desk, repetitive physical actions, heavy lifting, gardening, standing for long periods and sleeping on a soft mattress.

Emotional causes of stress are far more insidious. From the head, they create tension in the neck and shoulders and gradually invade the other body systems. Such stresses often result from interaction with other people, either at work or, at a deeper level, in personal relationships. They include anger, worry, fear, frustration, grief and unfulfilled emotions. In the Chinese view, disturbed or excessive emotions are the internal causes that lead to physical problems (see page 18).

The external causes of physical problems include the invasion of the body by environmental energies, such as heat, wind, cold, dryness and dampness. Other external

factors, such as poor diet, lack of exercise and insufficient sleep, worsen the effects of all of these. By identifying these factors, you may be able to modify your lifestyle to avoid them (see below).

LIFESTYLE ADVICE FOR THE MAINTENANCE OF HEALTH

- Eat a healthy, regular and well-balanced diet with no snacking between meals.
- Drink lots of water.
- Maintain regular sleep patterns with a minimum of seven hours of sleep.
- Take daily, moderate exercise, such as walking, swimming, yoga and qigong.
- Break long periods of sitting with frequent movement.
- Restrict alcohol consumption, and stop smoking or taking recreational drugs.
- Balance physical and mental work with rest, relaxation and exercise.
- Moderate your sexual activities.
- Never push your body to the extremes of endurance in work or exercise.
- Express your emotions.
- Wear warm clothing during cold weather to keep your trunk warm.
- Avoid excessive sunbathing.
- Use central heating or air conditioning with care.

TREATING SPORTS AND OTHER ACUTE INJURIES

Exercise and physical activity are vital to maintain health. Along with the recognized health benefits of sports, games and fitness training comes the risk of damage to muscles and joints. Sprains can occur almost anywhere on the body as the result of trauma.

Tui Na is a highly effective treatment for sports injuries, all of which cause qi and blood stagnation

> **CAUTION:** don't use ice on an injury unless there is bleeding. In TCM, warmth moves qi and blood to speed healing.

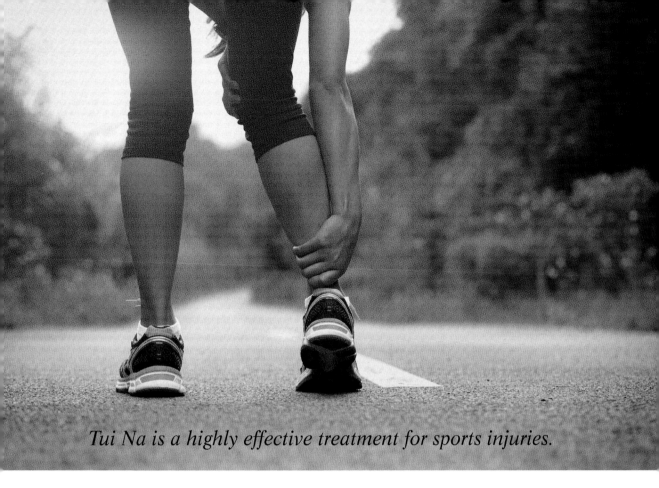

Tui Na is a highly effective treatment for sports injuries.

in the tissues, provided there are no broken bones or ruptured muscles and tendons. Spasming muscles, bursitis, damaged and inflamed tendons (tenosynovitis), overstretched ligaments, swelling (oedema) and bruising can all be treated successfully.

Begin the treatment as soon after the injury as possible. Identify the meridians that pass through the injured area (see chapter 3). Squeeze and knead along the affected meridians and focus on painful qi-points on and around the injury site with thumb pressure and kneading. Massage any ashi points around the injury – these are tender spots that may not exactly correspond with a qi-point. If the area is badly bruised, or if the skin is broken, use distal qi-points (see page 25) on the relevant meridians.

TREATING CHRONIC MUSCULOSKELETAL CONDITIONS

Osteoarthritis is a degenerative condition of bone, ligaments and cartilage. Rheumatoid arthritis is an inflammatory condition of the joints. In Chinese medicine these conditions are called 'bi syndrome'. It starts as qi and blood deficiency, which, on exposure to wind, cold, dampness or heat, leads to stagnation of qi and blood in the tissues. Tui Na excels in the treatment of chronic conditions like these.

FREQUENCY OF TUI NA TREATMENT

Tui Na treatment for specific conditions should be given daily for at least one week, then once a week until the pain has gone and mobility is restored.

THE TREATMENTS

Each treatment starts with a thorough soft tissue massage to prepare the tissues and joints, using steps from the relevant sections of the whole-body routine in chapter 5. Once your partner is warm and relaxed, start to work on the qi-points listed for the treatment, referring to the meridian illustrations and the captions that describe the positions of the points in chapter 3. Knead deeply on each of these qi-points for at least three minutes. For musculoskeletal points, the most effective local qi-points are shown in **bold**, while the distal points are used to enhance their effects. For internal conditions, points are divided into front and back qi-points. Finish by massaging along the meridians in that area. For maximum benefit, repeat the treatment daily, if possible, until symptoms subside.

Chronic and acute pain, including sports injuries

For the following, treat the recommended qi-points on the side of the body affected.

Neck and upper back pain

The trapezius and underlying muscles in the neck and shoulders easily become tense and knotted as a result of stress, causing a tight, heavy feeling and pain across the shoulders and neck affecting the gall bladder, bladder and small intestine meridians. With continued stress, muscles spasm, putting pressure on nerves, leading to headaches and pain in the arms and fingers. Chronic degenerative disease in the cervical spine, common in older people, also blocks qi and blood flow to cause pain.

Neck pain also results from trauma such as whiplash injuries from accidents or sport.

NECK PAIN TREATMENT

Apply Tui Na as described in chapter 5, Part One, steps 1–7. You can also treat the neck in the supine position, as shown in Part Seven, steps 9–11.

• For general tension in the neck and across the top of the shoulders, with or without pain, sports injury or whiplash:
LOCAL GB 20, GB 12, BL 10, GB 21, SJ 15, SI 13, SI 14, SI 15, BL 11
DISTAL SJ 3, SI 3, nailing (see page 63, single thumb kneading) SJ 1, SI 1, GB 39, GB 34, BL 60

• For pain or numbness down one side of the neck and radiating down one arm to the fingers, add:
DISTAL SI 3, SJ 3, SJ 5, LU 7, LI 4, LI 11
CAUTION: don't use LI 4 during pregnancy.

Lower back pain

Pain in the lumbar area is extremely debilitating. Acute lower back pain can be caused by muscle strain or nerve damage. As we age, arthritis may develop in the vertebrae and damage the intervertebral discs. This will reduce the mobility of the spine, which can result in severe, chronic pain. As tension develops, the muscles shorten and spasm. Resulting tension in the tissues puts pressure on the nerves, causing pain both locally and in the legs.

LOWER BACK PAIN TREATMENT

Apply Tui Na as described in chapter 5, Part Three, with emphasis on steps 2–8 and 12 (cupping); Part Four, steps 1–2 (buttocks) and 4–11 (back of leg); and Part Five, steps 3, 5, 6 and 11 (leg shake).

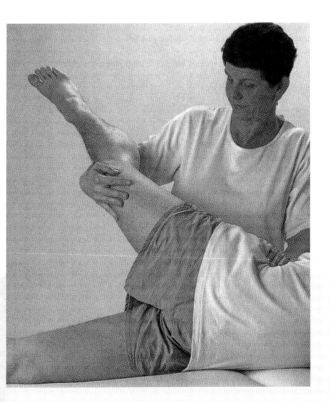

Manipulation of the lower back relieves pain from a rugby injury.

• For acute or chronic lumbar pain, with or without 'slipped disc':
LOCAL BL 22, BL 23, BL 24, BL 25, BL 26, BL 54
DISTAL BL 40, BL 60, BL 36, BL 37, BL 57

• For chronic lumbar pain due to weak kidney qi, choose from the above qi-points and focus on:
BL 23, K 3, K 13, R 4

• For chronic pain in the sacroiliac region:
LOCAL BL 23, BL 24, BL 25, BL 26, BL 27, BL 28, BL 32, BL 54
DISTAL BL 40, BL 60

Sciatica

Sciatica is chronic pain that radiates from the lower back/sacral region into the legs. It results from nerve damage, which can be triggered by a 'slipped disc', causing a nerve to be trapped. Nerves of the legs come from the spine. Damage to spinal nerves causes sciatica. It can be difficult to pinpoint the site of sciatic pain, which often seems to permeate the whole leg.

Sciatica has two components – inflammation of the spinal nerves and spasming leg muscles. Both of these cause pain. The first can be treated by massage on the lower back and the second by massage on the affected three leg yang meridians. It's important to palpate the three leg yang meridians – bladder, gall bladder and stomach – to identify which qi-points are painful.

SCIATICA TREATMENT

Apply Tui Na as described for the lower back and add side position and points shown above.

Your partner lies on their left side with a pillow supporting the head. The left leg is straight. Flex the right leg and draw it up in front so the thigh is almost at right angles to the body. Standing behind your partner and leaning over the right hip, elbow knead the buttock thoroughly. Focus on **GB 30** for at least two minutes with small, circular movements. Elbow knead **GB 29** and **BL 54** in the same way. Then squeeze with the whole hand, and knead with the heel of the hand down the flexed leg. Press and knead **GB 31** and **GB 34**.

Deep kneading of **GB 30** can be uncomfortable but relieves sciatica and hip pain. **BL 54** reinforces the benefits of **GB 30**.

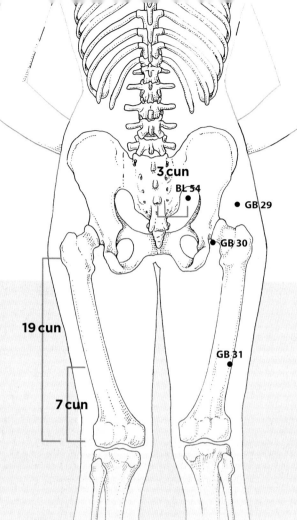

3 cun

BL 54

• GB 29

• GB 30

19 cun

GB 31

7 cun

MAIN QI-POINTS FOR LOWER BACK, HIP AND LEG MASSAGE
These are found on the gall bladder meridian (GB) and the bladder meridian (BL).

chronic. In extreme cases, this can turn into 'frozen shoulder', which is common in those over the age of fifty. In Chinese medicine, this is aggravated by exposure to wind, cold or dampness.

SHOULDER PAIN TREATMENT
Apply Tui Na as described in chapter 5, Part Two, steps 1–10 and 20; for top of shoulder, see Part One, steps 1–7.

• For pain in the deltoids and shoulder joint with or without immobility, due to acute soft tissue injury or joint degeneration:
LOCAL LI 15, jianqian, LI 14, SJ 14
DISTAL LI 11, LU 5, LI 4, SJ 5, GB 34
CAUTION: don't use LI 4 during pregnancy.

• For pain in scapular area and/or the back of the upper arm:
LOCAL SJ 14, SJ 10, SI 9, SI 10, SI 11, SI 12, SI 13, SI 14
DISTAL GB 34, SI 3

• For pain on top of the shoulder:
LOCAL GB 21, SJ 15, SI 14
DISTAL SJ 5, SJ 3

• For sciatica – lower back pain that radiates down one leg:
LOCAL BL 23, BL 24, BL 25, BL 26, GB 30, BL 54
DISTAL – GB meridian GB 31, GB 34, GB 39, GB 40
DISTAL – BL meridian BL 36, BL 37, BL 40, BL 57, BL 60
DISTAL – ST meridian ST 31, ST 34, ST 36

• For hip pain:
LOCAL GB 30, GB 29, BL 54
DISTAL GB 31, GB 34, GB 39, GB 40

Shoulder pain

There are a number of causes for shoulder pain, including all kinds of injury, inflammation and degeneration of tissues in the joint. Immobility often occurs when the condition becomes

Elbow pain

Repetitive strain injury of the elbow joint and surrounding tissues can result in conditions such as 'tennis elbow' and 'golfer's elbow'.

Wrists, in common with elbows, are subject to repetitive strain injuries and, in older people, arthritic conditions.

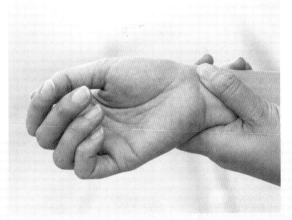

ELBOW PAIN TREATMENT

Apply Tui Na as described in chapter 5, Part Two, steps 11–14, followed by steps 9 and 10.

• For tennis elbow – pain in the outside of the elbow, often with extreme tenderness of the muscles overlying the upper third of the radius:
LOCAL LI 10, LI 11, LU 5 plus ashi points
(see pages 24 and 123)
DISTAL GB 34, SP 9, LI 4

• For golfer's elbow – pain in the inside of the joint and tenderness in the muscles on the inside of the upper forearm:
LOCAL H 3, P 3, SI 8 plus ashi points
(see pages 24 and 123)
DISTAL GB 34, SP 9, SI 3

Wrist pain

Wrists, in common with elbows, are subject to repetitive strain injuries, inflammation of the tendon sheaths (tenosynovitis) and, in older people, arthritic conditions. Carpal tunnel syndrome is a common wrist problem, where a nerve is compressed as it passes through the wrist, causing numbness or tingling in the fingers.

WRIST PAIN TREATMENT

Apply Tui Na as described in chapter 5, Part Two, steps 12–13 and 17–19 to massage and manipulate the hand and wrist.

LOCAL P7, H 7, LU 9, LI 5 and ashi points
(see pages 24 and 123)
DISTAL LU 7
Knead deeply around the wrist to stimulate all the qi-points on it. If the fingers are numb due to carpal tunnel syndrome, give particular attention to P 7.

Thumb pain

Thumb pain can be due to injury or arthritis.

THUMB PAIN TREATMENT

Apply Tui Na as described in chapter 5, Part Two, steps 13, 18 and 19. Rotate the thumb vigorously, pull it several times and roll it for thirty seconds between your palms.
LOCAL LI 4, LU 10 and any ashi points (see
pages 24 and 123)
CAUTION: don't use LI 4 during pregnancy.

Knee pain

Acute knee pain may be caused by a sprain or sports injury. Chronic pain can be due to sciatica, degeneration of the cartilage in the joint or inflamed ligaments.

If not caused by injury, most pain in the big toe, particularly in its basal joint, is probably the result of arthritis.

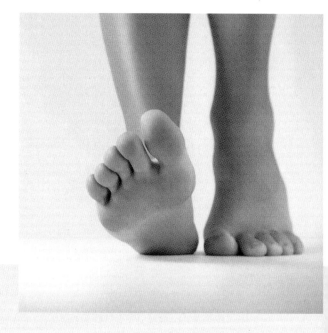

KNEE PAIN TREATMENT
Apply Tui Na as described in chapter 5, Part Five, steps 1, 2, 3, 7 and 8.

• For pain deep inside the knee joint caused by damaged cartilage or ligaments:
LOCAL ST 35 and xiyan Knead both points simultaneously and very deeply.
LOCAL ST 34, SP 10, ST 36, GB 34

• For pain caused by ligaments or tendons on the inner surface of the knee:
LOCAL SP 9, LV 8, SP 10, GB 34

• For pain caused by ligaments or tendons on the back of the knee:
LOCAL BL 40, K 10
DISTAL BL 37, BL 57

Ankle pain
'Twisted' ankles account for most ankle pain. In older people, weakness and chronic pain often results from arthritis.

ANKLE PAIN TREATMENT
Apply Tui Na as described in chapter 5, Part Five, step 12. Give a full foot massage, emphasizing the ankle rotation and deep kneading across the tendons.

• For acute or chronic pain within the ankle joints and general ankle weakness:
LOCAL LIV 4, GB 40, BL 60, ST 41, K 3, K 6

DISTAL GB 34, GB 39, SP 6, K7, GB 44 – press five times with nail.
CAUTION: don't use SP 6 during pregnancy.

• For sprain from ankle twisted outwards:
LOCAL GB 40, BL 60
DISTAL GB 34

• For sprain from ankle twisted inwards:
LOCAL K 3, K 6
DISTAL GB 34

• For inflammation of the Achilles tendon (squeeze and hack on the tendon):
LOCAL K 3, BL 60
DISTAL GB 34

Big toe pain
If not caused by injury, most pain in the big toe, particularly in its basal joint, is probably the result of arthritis.

BIG TOE PAIN TREATMENT
Apply Tui Na as described on page 121, steps 14 and 15, with several minutes of big toe rotations and pulls.
LOCAL LV 3, SP 4
DISTAL LI 4, LU 10

Common ailments

For the following, treat the recommended qi-points on both sides of the body.

Bronchial asthma

Asthma attacks are recurrent and can vary from mild to life-threatening. Attacks may be triggered by allergens such as pollen, dust, hair, feathers, smoke and even certain foods. Emotional stress often triggers asthma attack. To reduce the frequency of these attacks, massage qi-points to strengthen lung energies and calm the emotions.

BRONCHIAL ASTHMA TREATMENT

Apply Tui Na as described in chapter 5, Part One, steps 1, 3, 4 and 7; Part Six, steps 7 and 8; and Part Three, steps 1–8 (massage of the upper back).

• For the relief of symptoms:
FRONT POINTS R 17, LU 1, LU 2, LU 9, LU 7, LU 6, LU 5, P 6, P 8, LI 4, ST 40, ST 36
BACK POINTS BL 11, BL 12, BL 13, BL 23
CAUTION: don't use LI 4 during pregnancy.

Constipation

Sluggish action of the colon often results from a diet low in fibre, too little aerobic exercise or qi deficiency in old age.

CONSTIPATION TREATMENT

Apply Tui Na as described in chapter 5, Part Six, steps 1–10, and abdominal massage with emphasis on deep kneading around the periphery of the abdomen.
CAUTION: women who are pregnant should not be massaged on the abdomen.
FRONT POINTS ST 25, SP 15, K 16, R 6, R 4, ST 36, LI 4, GB 34, LIV 3
BACK POINTS BL 25, BL 20, BL 21
CAUTION: don't use LI 4 during pregnancy.

Diarrhoea

Acute diarrhoea resulting from contaminated food or water does not normally last for more than two or three days. If there is a sudden change of bowel habit to one of persistent diarrhoea, consult a doctor.

DIARRHOEA TREATMENT

Apply Tui Na as described in chapter 5, Part Six, steps 1–10 (abdominal massage).

FRONT POINTS ST 25, SP 15, R 12, SP 6, SP 9, ST 36, LI 11
BACK POINTS BL 25, BL 20, BL 21
• For vomiting accompanied by diarrhoea: **P 6**

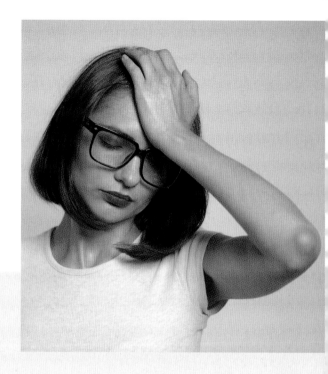

Irritable bowel syndrome – IBS

This condition is frequently stress-related. Symptoms include abdominal pain and indigestion, with diarrhoea or constipation – or both.

IBS TREATMENT

Apply Tui Na as described in chapter 5, Part Six, steps 1–10.

FRONT POINTS ST 25, SP 15, R 12, R 10, R 6, R 4, ST 36, SP 6, LI 4, LI 10, LI 11, LIV 3
BACK POINTS BL 20, BL 21, BL 25
CAUTION: don't use SP 6 or LI 4 during pregnancy.

Headaches and migraine

According to TCM, headaches and migraines are usually the result of disturbance to qi-flow in the yang meridians of the head – bladder, gall bladder and stomach. The most common headaches are tension headaches caused by emotions or excess alcohol. Migraines are severe, often accompanied by visual disturbances, nausea, vomiting and vertigo. If headaches are persistent and don't respond to Tui Na, consult a doctor.

HEADACHE AND MIGRAINE TREATMENT

Apply Tui Na as described in chapter 5, Part One, steps 1–7, followed by Part Seven, steps 1–11 (massage of the face and scalp).

• For headache at the base of the skull (occipital):
LOCAL GB 20, BL10, GB 21
DISTAL LI 4, BL 60, LIV 3
CAUTION: don't use LI 4 during pregnancy.

• For headache at the front of the head and/or ache around the eyes (frontal):
LOCAL GB 20, BL 2, GB 14, ST 8, yintang
DISTAL LI 4, GB 21, ST 41, ST 44
CAUTION: don't use LI 4 during pregnancy.

• For headache at the side of the head (lateral) and/or on the temples (temporal):
LOCAL taiyang, GB 20, GB 21, GB 8
DISTAL LI 4, SJ 3, SJ 5
CAUTION: don't use LI 4 during pregnancy.

• For headache at the top of the head (vertex):
LOCAL DU 20
DISTAL LIV 3, LI 4

• For migraine with nausea and vomiting:
LOCAL P 6, ST 36, LIV 3, GB 20

Use other points according to where the pain manifests, as above.

In TCM, headaches and migraines are usually the result of disturbance to qi-flow in the yang meridians of the head.

Other common conditions

Enlarged prostate gland

Difficulty in passing urine.

FRONT POINTS R 3, R 4, K 3, K 7, SP 6
BACK POINTS BL 23, BL 32

High blood pressure – hypertension

FRONT POINTS LIV 3, K 1, K 3, K 7, ST 36, P 6, LI 11, DU 20
BACK POINTS GB 20

Blood pressure tends to fall during Tui Na treatment, whether or not there is high blood pressure.

Heart problems

FRONT POINTS P 6, H 7
BACK POINTS BL 15, BL 14

Infertility

FRONT POINTS R 4, R 6, ST 25, ST 29, P 6, SP 6, K 3, K 1
BACK POINTS BL 23, BL 32

Premenstrual tension – PMT

FRONT POINTS R 6, R 4, SP 6, LIV 3, LI 4
BACK POINTS GB 20, GB 11
CAUTION: don't use SP 6 or LI 4 during pregnancy.

Insomnia

According to TCM, insomnia is frequently a problem related to the substance shen (see page 16). It results in difficulty getting to sleep because of an active mind, shallow sleep disturbed by dreams, or waking in the night and being unable to get back to sleep. Tui Na for the neck, shoulder, back and face are particularly effective for insomnia treatment.

INSOMNIA TREATMENT

Apply Tui Na as described in chapter 5, Part Seven, steps 1–11.

FRONT POINTS H 7, P 6, P 7, P 8, yintang, K 1, R 4, SP 6, ST 36, LIV 3, DU 20
BACK POINTS BL 15, BL 14
CAUTION: don't use SP 6 during pregnancy.

Emotional stress

Emotions such as anxiety, worry and frustration all cause stress. They can be treated by calming the

Tui Na massage for children under the age of six is widely practised in China.

shen (see page 16) and reducing stagnation in the liver and gall bladder meridians.

EMOTIONAL TREATMENT
This covers anxiety, worry, anger, frustration and sadness.

FRONT POINTS yintang, taiyang, DU 20, GB 13, P 6, P 7, P 8, H 7, LIV 3, SP 6, K3, K1
BACK POINTS GB 20, GB 21
CAUTION: don't use SP 6 during pregnancy.

Runny or blocked nose, hay fever and sinusitis
Sinusitis is an inflammation of the facial sinuses, resulting in a blocked nose and pressure around the eyes. Hay fever symptoms include runny or blocked nose, sneezing and red, itchy eyes.

RUNNY OR BLOCKED NOSE, HAY FEVER AND SINUSITIS TREATMENT
Apply Tui Na as described in chapter 5, Part One, steps 5–6, and Part Seven, steps 1, 3, 4 and 5.

FRONT POINTS LI 20, yintang, BL 2, LI 4, LU 5, LU 7, LU 1, LU 2
BACK POINTS BL 11, BL 12, BL 13
CAUTION: don't use LI 4 during pregnancy.

Eye problems
REFRESHING EYES AND IMPROVING VISION TREATMENT
Eyesight depends on a good supply of qi. All the following local points boost eye health and can also improve some conditions such as twitching eyelids and sore, red or shadowy eyes.

FRONT POINTS BL 2, SJ 23, GB 1, ST 1, GB 14, taiyang, LIV 3, GB 43
BACK POINTS GB 20

Hearing problems
POOR HEARING, BLOCKED EARS, MILD TINNITUS TREATMENT
FRONT POINTS SJ 21, SI 19, GB 2, GB 8, ST 7
BACK POINTS GB 12

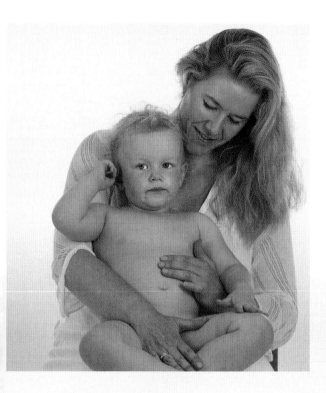

Tui Na for infants

Paediatric Tui Na massage is a specialized branch of massage for children under the age of six and is widely practised in China. In young children the meridian system is delicate and still in the process of development. Paediatric Tui Na uses some extra points that are not used on adults, particularly on the hands, accessing the energies of the internal organs through the fingers. Each of the five fingers is linked with one of the yin organs. All the qi-points and soft tissue techniques in this book can be used safely on young children to enhance full physical and mental development and boost the immune system. Use light pressure at first, increasing it gradually as the child adapts.

Three effective techniques for common conditions are described here, one of which is a special hand technique for under-fives.

Rubbing the abdomen
Use the palm of the hand to rub clockwise at least fifty times around the abdomen.

BENEFITS
Excellent for restlessness. Strengthens the spleen and stomach and promotes healthy functioning of the digestive tract.

Stroking the eyebrows – meigong
Using your middle fingers, start at **BL 2** and stroke outwards towards **SJ 23**. Repeat fifty times.

BENEFITS
The technique – known as meigong – is powerfully calming, promotes healthy eyes and stimulates brain development. It also treats colds and coughs.

Rubbing around the neibagua
The neibagua is a circular area around qi-point **P 8**. A good time to use this technique is just before bedtime. Using very small circular movements, knead **P 8** at least fifty times. Now rub clockwise the area around **P 8** – the neibagua – making between fifty and one hundred circles, and repeat on the other hand.

BENEFITS
Regulates the six yin and six yang organs and balances the qi energies between them to boost immunity and brain development. Soothes a baby who has colic.

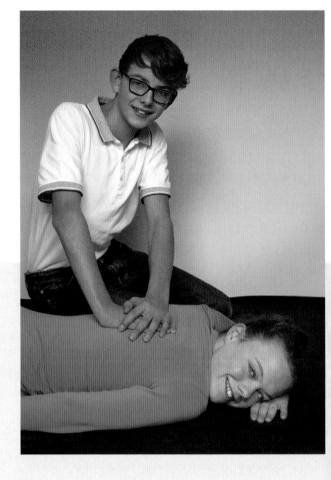

Tui Na in adolescence

Adolescence is the period of physical, mental and emotional change and maturation that marks the change from childhood to adulthood. Many adolescents are taking exams and having to make important career choices, which can cause anxiety, worry and frustration.

The typical physical problems of adolescence are usually due to hormonal imbalance and lifestyle.

Tui Na can help the body recover from living life in the fast lane, such as late nights, erratic and unhealthy meals and lack of sleep.

TREATMENT FOR ADOLESCENTS

Have fun trying out different Tui Na techniques and finding the qi-points. Kneading along the bladder meridian and massaging the neck and shoulders relieves tension. Use the shu points on the bladder meridian of the back (see page 26) to strengthen the organs. See elsewhere in this chapter for treatments for insomnia, anxiety and other conditions.

Tui Na can help the body recover from living life in the fast lane, such as late nights, erratic and unhealthy meals and lack of sleep.

Squeezing the top of the shoulders improves qi and blood flow, removing any stagnation to create a feeling of well-being.

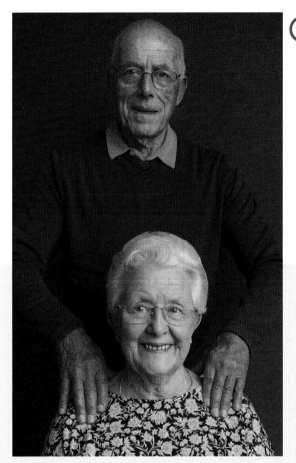

Tui Na in later years

According to Chinese theory, the problems associated with ageing are due to both qi and blood deficiency and stagnation as we grow older. The ageing process cannot be stopped, but with Tui Na you can feel good and reasonably pain free. People in their late eighties can enjoy Tui Na just as much as those in their thirties. When massaging an elderly person, bear in mind that joints become less mobile with age, and lying face down may be difficult, so you may have to give treatments in other positions. Be aware that the soft tissues are often tender and can bruise very easily, and that older people may have less body fat and less 'padding' on the bones. They may also have osteoporosis.

TREATMENT IN LATER YEARS
The neck, shoulders, arms and back should be massaged unless specifically contraindicated (see page 62).

Squeezing the top of the shoulders improves qi and blood flow, removing any stagnation to create a feeling of well-being.

A gentle arm rotation loosens an arthritic shoulder joint, relieving pain and increasing flexibility.

TUI NA SELF-TREATMENT

Tui Na identifies healthcare qi-points that are particularly effective for stimulating qi and blood flow, thus maintaining balance between the organ functions and inhibiting the onset of stagnation. For general good health, you can give yourself a daily workout, kneading the healthcare qi-points listed below. The whole-body routine works on all these points. The positions of these points are shown and described on the meridian illustrations on pages 32–59.

Daily healthcare qi-points for well-being

For general well-being, press and knead these healthcare qi-points at least daily.

- Start on the head and knead:
  DU 20, yintang

- Use the middle and/or index fingers of both hands to knead:
  BL 2, SJ 23, GB 13, GB 14, taiyang, GB 8
  LI 20, SI 19, SJ 17
  GB 20, BL 10
  GB 21 one side at a time

- Working on each arm in turn, use the thumb and middle and index fingers to knead:
  LI 15 and **SJ 14** together
  LI 11 and **H 3** together
  SJ 5 and **P 6** together

- Thumb knead each hand in turn and then shake your wrists vigorously, using:
  H 7, P 7, LU 9, P 8, LI 4, SJ 3

- Nail press and then pull each finger, using:
  LU 11, LI 1, SJ 1, SI 1, H 9, P 9

- Lying on your back, knead:
  R 17, R 12, R 10, R 6, R 4, ST 25, SP 15

- Put both your hands behind your waist and thumb knead:
  BL 23

- Using both your knuckles, knead vigorously:
  GB 30

- Using the thumbs of both hands, knead the inner leg qi-points:
  SP 9, SP 6, K 3, K 6

- Using the index, middle and fourth fingers to do circular kneading with both hands, knead the outer leg qi-points:
  ST 36, GB 34, ST 40

- If you can reach your feet, knead each foot separately, using:
  LIV 3, K 1, SP 3, SP 4
  CAUTION: don't use LI 4 or SP 6 during pregnancy.

If you have a like-minded partner, you should have all the back shu points, from **BL 11** to **BL 26**, kneaded every day.

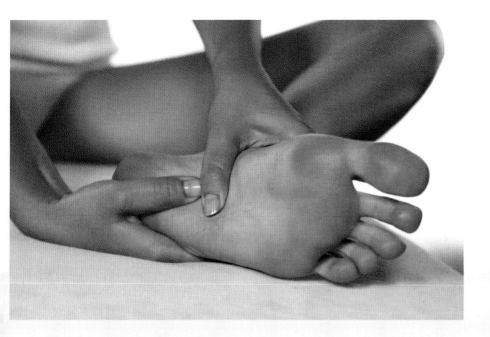

Everyone can benefit from a daily Tui Na session.

Daily Tui Na – self-pummelling the meridians

Everyone can benefit from a daily Tui Na session. The best method is to pummel all the accessible parts of the body and knead the essential qi-points. If you make this a daily routine, you will boost your 'feel-good' factor and slow down the ageing process.

Start pummelling with your right hand down the inside of your left arm to the hand and then up the outside. Repeat several times. Then work with your left hand on the right arm. Support your right elbow with your left hand as you pummel across the top of the left shoulder, reaching **GB 21**. Repeat on the other side.

Using both hands, pummel the front of the chest, particularly in the region of the qi-points **LU 1** and **LU 2**. From standing, bend forwards and pummel down both sides of the back and buttocks to stimulate the bladder meridian and **GB 30**. Then, using the heels of both hands, vigorously rub **BL 23** to stimulate the kidney.

Remaining in the forward-leaning position, move the legs apart and pummel down the outside and then up the inside of both the legs simultaneously. Lift one leg onto a chair, as high as is comfortable, and pummel with both hands up and down. Repeat for the other leg.

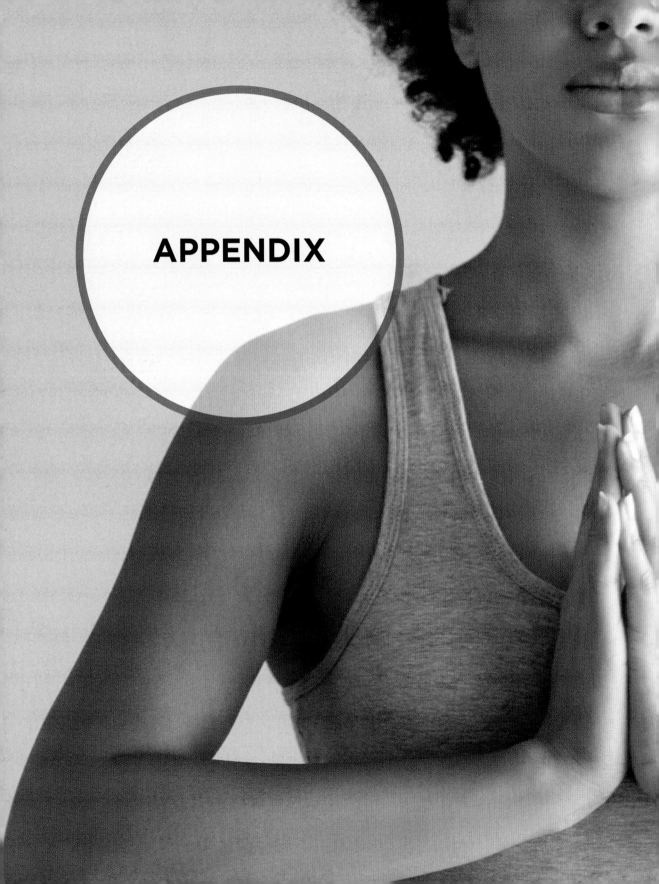

APPENDIX

The fixed cun measurements

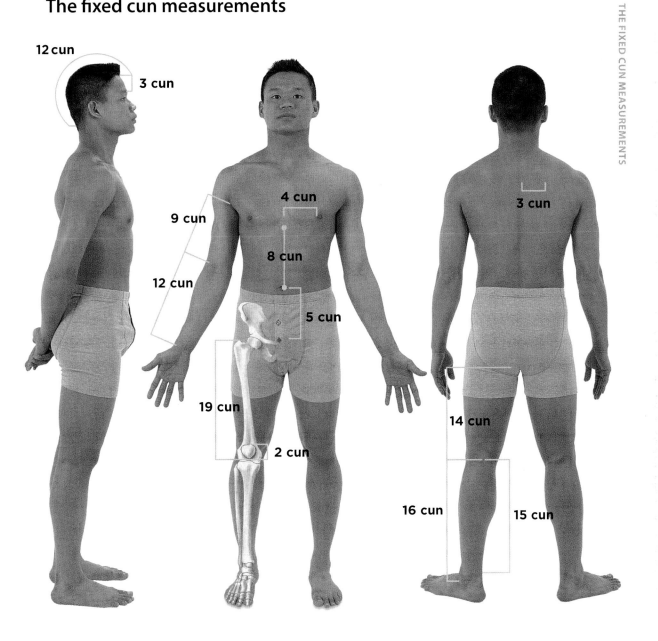

12 cun

3 cun

4 cun

9 cun

8 cun

12 cun

5 cun

3 cun

19 cun

2 cun

14 cun

16 cun

15 cun

Elbow crease to wrist crease **12 cun**
Elbow crease to armpit crease **9 cun**
Lateral knee to lateral ankle **16 cun**
Medial knee to medial ankle bone **15 cun**
Navel to pubic bone **5 cun**
Navel to sternoxiphoid tip **8 cun**
Centre sternum to nipple **4 cun**

Centre spine to medial scapula **3 cun**
Great trochanter to side knee crease **19 cun**
Height of patella **2 cun**
Buttock crease to knee crease **14 cun**
Eyebrow to hairline **3 cun**
Front hairline to back hairline **12 cun**

The muscles

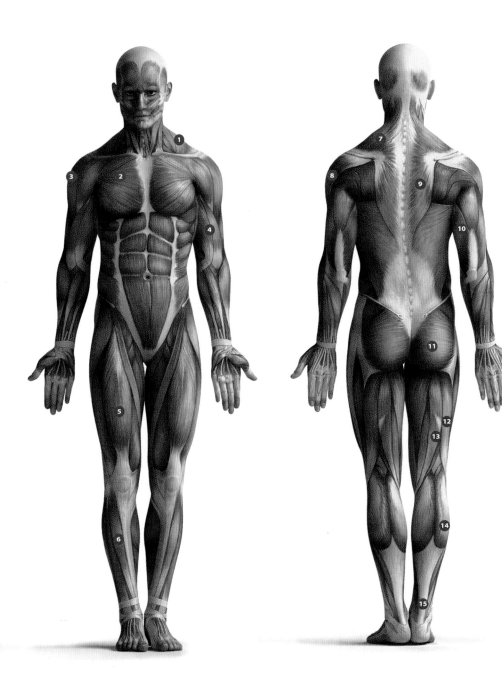

1 trapezius
2 pectoral
3 deltoid
4 biceps
5 quadriceps
6 tibialis anterior
7 trapezius
8 deltoid
9 rhomboid
10 triceps
11 gluteus maximus
12 biceps femoris
13 semitendinosus
14 gastrocnemius
15 Achilles tendon

The bones

To find back shu points (see page 26), use the following landmarks. To locate cervical vertebra seven (C 7) look for the most prominent vertebra on the base of the neck. Place your finger on its spinous process, and ask your partner to turn their head from side to side. If the vertebra moves slightly, it's C 7. The one below it, thoracic one (T 1), doesn't move. BL 11 is level with the lower end of the spinous process of T 1, which feels like a small gap. To locate BL 25, feel for the highest point on the ilium on the lower back – BL 25 is level with this and with the lower end of the spinous process of lumbar vertebra four. BL 26 is in the next space down, just above the sacrum. To find BL 23, slide up two vertebrae and check this by feeling for the lowest ribs. BL 23 is level with these.

1 collarbone
2 humerus
3 intercostal space
4 radius
5 ulna
6 pubic bone
7 metacarpal bones
8 femur
9 patella – kneecap
10 fibula
11 tibia
12 external malleolus
13 internal malleolus
14 metatarsal bones
15 occipital bone
16 cervical vertebrae (7)
17 acromion
18 scapula
19 scapular spine

20 thoracic vertebrae (12)
21 spinous process of vertebrae
22 lumbar vertebrae (5)
23 iliac crest
24 ilium
25 sacrum
26 coccyx
27 ischium
28 head of fibula

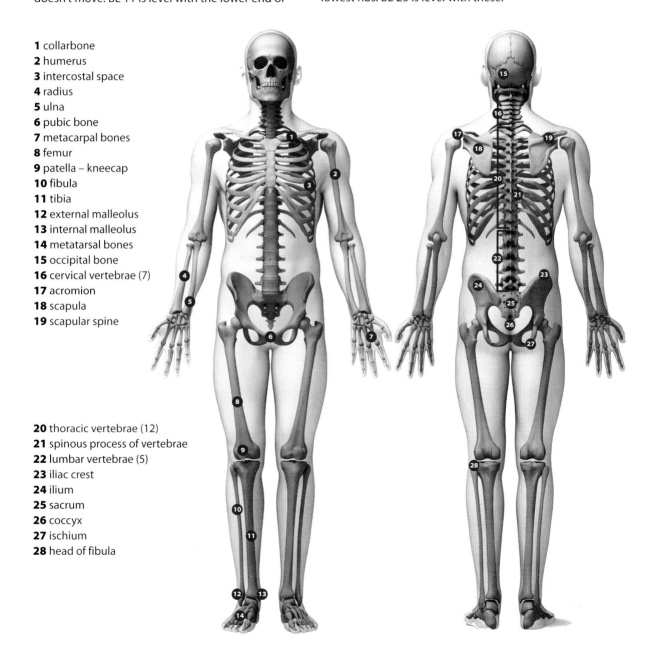

GLOSSARY

Achilles tendon tendon that connects the calf muscles to the heel bone (see page 154)

acute describes a sudden, intense condition that may be of short duration

adipose fatty

bilateral two-sided

bursitis inflammation of a bursa, a fluid-filled sac that acts as padding for the joints

cartilage gristle on the surfaces of bones in the joints

cervical of the neck

chafe to rub the skin (see page 68)

chiropractice treatment of disorders through manipulation, especially of the spine

chronic describes a persistent and debilitating condition

connective tissue cells supporting and connecting organs, also ligaments and tendons

cun a non-standard measurement (see pages 24–5 and 153)

cupping a percussive technique (see page 70)

deltoid the thick muscle on the outer edge of the shoulder (see page 154)

du a meridian (see pages 29 and 59)

eczema skin inflammation with scaly, itching or burning lesions

fibrositis inflammation of fibrous tissue, in particuiar around muscles

fibula the thin outer bone of the lower leg (see page 155)

hack to strike with the edge of the hand (see page 70)

hamstring the tendon at the back of the knee

humerus the upper arm bone (see page 155)

iliosacral describes the region joining the sacrum and ilium (see page 155)

ligament fibre linking bone and cartilage

lumbago pain in the lower back

lumbar of the region between the lowest ribs and the hipbones

mastoid process a bony, downward projection from the skull just behind the ear

meridian a channel through which qi flows

metacarpal hand bone between the wrist and the knuckles (see page 155)

midline the central line of the body, viewed from the front or back

neuralgia severe pain along one or more nerves

occipital of the back of the head or skull

osteoarthritis degenerative condition of the joints, creating pain and stiffness

osteopathy a system of healing based on manipulation, particularly of the bones

osteoporosis a condition where the bones become porous and brittle, due to calcium loss

palmar of the palm of the hand

pectoral large chest muscle that moves the shoulder and upper arm (see page 154)

percussion striking or hitting (see page 70)

pericardium an organ closely linked to the heart

pluck to push across muscled tissue (see page 67)

PMT premenstrual tension; also called premenstrual syndrome

prolapse sinking of an organ or body part from its normal position

psoriasis skin disease with reddish, scaly, itching patches

pummel to strike the skin with loose fists (see page 71)

qi vital energy or life force, which flows in meridians

qi-point point on a meridian where qi can be manipulated

radius the outer bone of the lower arm (see page 155)

ren a meridian (see pages 29 and 58)

rheumatoid arthritis a chronic disease of the musculoskeletal system, with joint inflammation, swelling and pain

rhinitis inflammation of the nose membranes

rhomboid muscle between the spine and the shoulder (see page 154)

sacrum wedge-shaped bone at the base of the spine (see page 155)

scapula the triangular back shoulder bone (see page 155)

sciatica neuralgia of the sciatic nerve, which runs down the leg

sinusitis inflammation of the sinuses

spasming describe muscles that are overcontracting

spinous process the outward bony protrusion of a vertebra (see page 155)

tendon fibrous tissue joining muscle to bone

thoracic of the thorax, the area between the neck and the lumbar region

tinnitus ringing in the ears

trapezius flat triangular muscle on the side of the back, shoulders and neck (see page 154)

ulna the inner, longer bone of the lower arm (see page 155)

yin and **yang** two aspects of the underlying principle of Chinese philosophy (see page 17)

RESOURCES

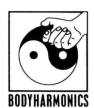

BODYHARMONICS®
54 Flecker's Drive
Cheltenham GL51 5BD
Tel: +44 (0)1242 582168

www.bodyharmonics.co.uk
e-mail: maria@bodyharmonics.co.uk

TRAINING COURSES

Maria Mercati's
- **Tui Na Chinese massage course**
- **Acupuncture**

There are very few qualified Tui Na therapists in the West. For a register of qualified Tui Na and Acupuncture practitioners in the UK, go to: **www.acupuncture-acutherapy.co.uk**

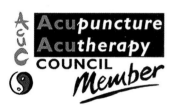

FURTHER RESOURCES

The Thai Massage Manual by Maria Mercati
Shows acupressure points used on different parts of the body. DVD to accompany book.

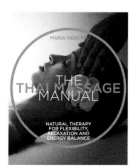

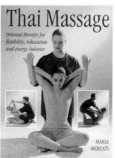

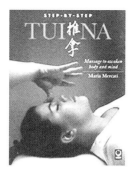

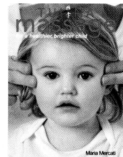

TUI NA DVDs

- *Step-by-Step Tui Na*
  Clearly demonstrates the techniques, the routine and where to stand in relation to your partner. Excellent companion to the book.
- *Tui Na Massage for a Healthier, Brighter Child*

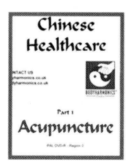

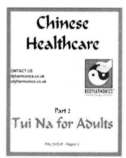

SIX CHINESE HEALTHCARE DVDs

Maria Mercati's series of DVDs on Chinese healthcare as practised and filmed in Chinese hospitals.
- Acupuncture
- Tui Na for Adults
- Tui Na for Children
- Food and Herbs
- Qigong and Tai Chi
- Teach Yourself Five Animal Qigong

INDEX

Page numbers in **bold** refer to
main text entries

EDDISON BOOKS LIMITED
Creative Consultant **Nick Eddison**
Managing Editor **Tessa Monina**
Production **Sarah Rooney & Cara Clapham**
Proofreader **Nikky Twyman**
Indexer **Marie Lorimer**

Designed and edited by **3redcars.co.uk**

Cover John Hytch

ShutterStockphoto.Inc 2 Minerva Studio; 6 feiyuezhangjie; 25 tl, tc Alexey Boldin; 25 tr Zemler; 30 Triff; 36 fluke samed; 42 Vasilev Evgenii; 48 mexrix; 52 r.classen; 88 Yuganov Konstantin; 98 Image Point Fr; 106 puhhha; 114 milanzeremski; 122 Image Point Fr; 128 Maridav; 137 lzf; 141 I'm friday; 142 FotoDuets; 144 Borysevych.com; 151 Vladimir Gjorgiev; 152 LStockStudio; 155 Sebastian Kaulitzki

Thinkstock 84 b-d-s; 154 cosmin4000

147, 148, 149 Gina Mercati; 153 Sue Atkinson

All illustrations on pages 90, 91, 95, 101, 102, 108, 109, 112, 113, 116, 121, 124, 130, 131 Paul Oakley

All other images John Hytch